Contents

INTRODUCTION

Welcome to the High-Fat, Zero-Carb, Zero-Sugar diet! In this book, we will explore the benefits of this diet, including weight loss, improved blood sugar control, and increased energy. We will also discuss the potential challenges of maintaining this diet long-term and provide practical tips and strategies for success.

We will begin by discussing the basic principles of the High-Fat, Zero-Carb, Zero-Sugar diet, including what foods to eat and avoid. We will explore the benefits of incorporating low-carb vegetables into meals and snacks, as well as the importance of meal planning and recipe modifications.

Throughout, we will provide sample meal plans and recipes for breakfast, lunch, dinner, and snacks, and discuss how to modify recipes to fit your dietary needs. We will also address social situations and offer tips for incorporating occasional treats while staying on track.

By the end of this book, you will have a solid understanding of the High-Fat, Zero-Carb, Zero-Sugar diet, and the tools you need to successfully maintain this diet for long-term health and wellness.

CHAPTER ONE

THE H0 DIET: AN OVERVIEW

Definition of the High-fat, Zero-Carb, Zero-Sugar diet (H0)

The High-fat, Zero-Carb, Zero-Sugar diet, also known as the "H0 diet", is a dietary approach that emphasizes a high intake of healthy fats, moderate protein intake, and minimal to no intake of carbohydrates and sugars. The H0 diet is based on the idea that consuming high levels of carbohydrates and sugars can lead to spikes in blood sugar and insulin levels, which can contribute to a variety of health issues such as weight gain, inflammation, and insulin resistance.

By drastically reducing carbohydrate and sugar intake, the H0 diet encourages the body to enter a metabolic state called ketosis, where it starts to burn fat for energy instead of carbohydrates. This can lead to significant weight loss, improved blood sugar control, increased energy levels, and reduced inflammation.

The H0 diet typically includes foods such as healthy fats like olive oil, coconut oil, and avocado, as well as protein sources like meat, fish, and eggs. It also includes low-carb vegetables like leafy greens, broccoli, and cauliflower. Foods that are high in carbohydrates and sugars, such as bread, pasta, sugar, and processed snacks, are avoided or eliminated completely.

The emphasis on high-fat foods and avoidance of carbohydrates and sugars

The H0 diet emphasizes the consumption of high-fat foods while avoiding carbohydrates and sugars. The rationale behind this dietary approach is that by drastically reducing carbohydrate and sugar intake, the body is forced to use fat as its primary source of energy instead of glucose. This process, known as ketosis, is believed to have several health benefits, including weight loss, improved blood sugar control, and increased energy levels.

In the H0 diet, the emphasis is on consuming healthy fats such as avocados, nuts and seeds, coconut oil, olive oil, and fatty fish like salmon. These foods are nutrient-dense and provide the body with important vitamins and minerals. On the other hand, carbohydrates and sugars are largely avoided, including foods such as bread, pasta, rice, potatoes, sugar, and processed foods that contain added sugars.

While the H0 diet may seem extreme, it has gained popularity in recent years due to its reported health benefits. However, it is important to note that this diet is not for everyone and should only be undertaken under the guidance of a healthcare professional. Additionally, individuals who choose to follow this diet may need to supplement their intake with certain vitamins and minerals to ensure that they are meeting their nutritional needs.

The goal of the H0 diet: to induce ketosis and burn fat for energy.

The goal of the H0 diet is to induce a metabolic state called ketosis, which occurs when the body burns fat for energy instead of carbohydrates. This is achieved by drastically reducing carbohydrate and sugar intake and increasing fat consumption.

Normally, the body uses glucose, derived from carbohydrates, as its primary source of energy. However, when carbohydrate intake is limited, the body turns to stored fat for energy, which is broken down into molecules called ketones. These ketones can then be used as an alternative source of fuel for the brain and body.

By maintaining a state of ketosis, the body can burn fat for energy, which can lead to weight loss and other health benefits. Additionally, ketosis has been shown to have positive effects on blood sugar regulation, cholesterol levels, and even brain function.

However, it is important to note that the H0 diet is not suitable for everyone and should be approached with caution. It may not be appropriate for those with certain medical conditions or those who are pregnant or breastfeeding. It is always best to consult with a healthcare professional before starting any new diet or making significant changes to your diet.

Potential Benefits of the H0 Diet

Weight loss and appetite suppression

Weight loss and appetite suppression are two significant benefits of the H0 diet. This diet has been shown to help individuals lose weight, even in the absence of calorie counting or portion control. By limiting carbohydrate intake, the body is forced to burn fat for energy instead of glucose from carbohydrates, leading to weight loss.

Moreover, the high-fat content of the H0 diet can help suppress appetite and reduce food cravings. Fats take longer to digest than carbohydrates, which can help individuals feel fuller for longer periods of time. This can lead to a reduction in overall food intake, resulting in weight loss.

Additionally, the H0 diet can have a positive effect on hormones involved in hunger and satiety, such as insulin and leptin. By reducing carbohydrate intake, the body produces less insulin, which can help prevent insulin resistance and improve insulin sensitivity. Leptin, a hormone that regulates appetite, can also be positively affected by the H0 diet. Studies have shown that this diet can increase leptin sensitivity, which can help reduce food intake and promote weight loss.

Improvements in blood lipid levels, blood pressure, and blood glucose control

In addition to weight loss and appetite suppression, the H0 diet has been shown to have several other health benefits. One of these benefits is improvements in blood lipid levels, blood pressure, and blood glucose control.

Studies have found that following the H0 diet can lead to a reduction in triglycerides and an increase in HDL ("good") cholesterol, which can help lower the risk of heart disease. The diet has also been shown to lower blood pressure, which is another risk factor for heart disease.

Furthermore, the H0 diet has been shown to improve blood glucose control in people with type 2 diabetes. By limiting carbohydrates and sugars, the body is forced to use fat for energy, which can lead to a reduction in insulin resistance and improved blood sugar levels. This can be especially beneficial for those with type 2 diabetes who struggle to control their blood sugar through medication alone.

Overall, the H0 diet may have significant health benefits beyond just weight loss and appetite suppression, including improvements in blood lipid levels, blood pressure, and blood glucose control.

Potential reduction of inflammation

The H0 diet may potentially reduce inflammation in the body. Inflammation is the body's natural response to injury or infection, but chronic inflammation can lead to various health problems, including heart disease, diabetes, and cancer. Carbohydrates and sugar can trigger an inflammatory response in the body, while healthy fats have been shown to have anti-inflammatory effects.

The H0 diet emphasizes whole, nutrient-dense foods such as grass-fed meats, wild-caught fish, healthy fats, and low-carb vegetables. These foods are high in anti-inflammatory nutrients such as omega-3 fatty acids, antioxidants, and phytochemicals. Additionally, the reduction of carbohydrates and sugars in the diet may help to lower insulin levels, which can also reduce inflammation in the body.

Several studies have found that the H0 diet may reduce markers of inflammation in the body. For example, one study in overweight women found that following an H0 diet for 12 weeks led to significant reductions in markers of inflammation, including C-reactive protein and interleukin-6. Another study in patients with type 2 diabetes found that following an H0 diet for six months led to significant reductions in several markers of inflammation, including tumor necrosis factor-alpha and interleukin-6.

While more research is needed to fully understand the anti-inflammatory effects of the H0 diet, these findings suggest that it may be a promising dietary approach for reducing inflammation and improving overall health.

Possible benefits for brain function and cancer risk reduction

There is some evidence to suggest that the H0 diet may have potential benefits for brain function and reducing the risk of certain types of cancer.

> **Brain Function:**

The brain relies on glucose as its primary fuel source, but in the absence of glucose from carbohydrates, the body can use ketones derived from fat as an alternative fuel source. This is known as ketosis, and some studies suggest that it may have neuroprotective effects and improve cognitive function. In fact, the ketogenic diet was initially developed in the 1920s as a treatment for epilepsy and has been found to be effective in reducing seizures in some patients.

> **Cancer Risk Reduction:**

There is also some evidence to suggest that the H0 diet may reduce the risk of certain types of cancer. Cancer cells are known to rely on glucose as a fuel source, and some studies have found that reducing carbohydrate intake may slow the growth of cancer cells. Additionally, the H0 diet may help to reduce inflammation, which is thought to play a role in the development of some types of cancer.

Potential benefits for athletes in endurance performance and muscle recovery

The H0 diet may also have potential benefits for athletes, particularly those engaged in endurance sports. This is because it can help the body become more efficient at burning fat for fuel, which can lead to increased endurance performance.

Additionally, the H0 diet may also aid in muscle recovery after exercise. Some studies have shown that a high-fat diet can help reduce inflammation and promote muscle repair and growth.

Mechanism of Action

Shifting the body's metabolism to rely on fat for fuel.

The H0 diet is designed to shift the body's metabolism from relying on glucose (sugar) for fuel to relying on fat for fuel. By drastically reducing carbohydrate intake, the body is forced to break down stored fat into molecules called ketones, which can be used as a source of energy. This metabolic state is called ketosis.

While in ketosis, the body is more efficient at burning fat for fuel, which can lead to increased weight loss and improved body composition. In addition, some proponents of the H0 diet argue that burning fat for fuel may provide more sustained energy throughout the day, without the energy crashes that can occur with a high-carbohydrate diet.

Production of ketones and their anti-inflammatory properties

When following the H0 diet, the body shifts its metabolism to rely on fat for fuel instead of carbohydrates. As a result, the liver produces molecules called ketones, which are a type of fuel that the body can use in place of glucose.

One of the potential benefits of producing ketones is their anti-inflammatory properties. Inflammation is a natural response to injury or infection, but chronic inflammation can contribute to a wide range of health problems, including heart disease, diabetes, and cancer.

Ketones may help reduce inflammation by inhibiting the production of certain inflammatory molecules in the body, such as cytokines and chemokines. Additionally, ketones may activate pathways in the body that promote antioxidant defense, which can help reduce oxidative stress and inflammation.

Studies have shown that the H0 diet can reduce markers of inflammation in the body, such as C-reactive protein (CRP), which is a well-established marker of inflammation and a risk factor for cardiovascular disease. In one study, participants following a H0 diet had significant reductions in CRP levels compared to a control group.

Overall, the production of ketones and their anti-inflammatory properties are potential mechanisms by which the H0 diet may provide health benefits beyond just weight loss.

Potential Drawbacks

Challenges of adhering to a diet that requires a dramatic shift in eating habits.

The H0 diet can be a challenging diet to follow because it requires a significant shift in eating habits. For many people, this may mean giving up foods they are used to eating regularly, such as bread, pasta, rice, and sugary treats.

Another challenge is the need to carefully track macronutrient intake. To maintain the state of ketosis required for the diet to be effective, individuals must consume a high amount of fat, a moderate amount of protein, and very few carbohydrates. This means that meal planning, and preparation can be time-consuming and require a lot of attention to detail.

Eating out and social situations can also be challenging, as many restaurant meals and social events may not fit within the parameters of the H0 diet. This can make it difficult to stick to the diet when dining out with friends or attending parties or gatherings.

Finally, some people may experience side effects when first starting the diet, such as fatigue, headaches, and constipation, as the body adjusts to the new eating pattern. These side effects usually subside after a few days or weeks, but they can make it challenging to stick to the diet in the beginning.

Despite these challenges, many people have found success with the H0 diet by carefully planning their meals, finding support from others, and focusing on the many health benefits that can come from following this type of eating pattern.

Concerns about high protein intake and kidney function

There is some concern about the potential impact of a high-protein diet on kidney function. The kidneys play a crucial role in filtering waste products from the blood and excreting them in urine. Some studies suggest that a diet high in protein may increase the workload on the kidneys, potentially leading to long-term damage or dysfunction.

However, the evidence linking high-protein diets to kidney damage is mixed, and more research is needed to fully understand the relationship between protein intake and kidney health. It is worth noting that most studies that have found a link between high protein intake and kidney damage have been conducted on individuals with preexisting kidney disease or impaired kidney function.

For healthy individuals, moderate to high protein intake is generally considered safe and may even have some health benefits. It is important to consume a variety of protein sources and not rely solely on animal-based proteins, which can be high in saturated fat and cholesterol. Plant-based sources of protein, such as beans, lentils, and tofu, can be excellent choices for a high-protein, low-carb diet like the H0 diet.

Before starting any new diet, it is important to consult with a healthcare provider to ensure that it is safe and appropriate for your individual needs and health status. This is especially true for diets that require a significant shift in eating habits.

A healthcare provider can assess your medical history, current health status, and any medications you may be taking to determine if the H0 diet is safe for you to try. They can also help you create a plan to ensure that you are meeting your nutrient needs and avoiding any potential health risks associated with the diet, such as nutrient deficiencies or kidney problems.

Additionally, a healthcare provider can monitor your progress and provide guidance on how to adjust your diet if necessary. This can help ensure that you are following the diet safely and effectively, and that you are achieving the desired health outcomes.

Explanation of why traditional low-fat diets don't work.

Brief history of low-fat diets as the recommended approach to weight loss and overall health

In the 1970s, a series of studies and reports suggested that a diet high in fat and cholesterol was linked to heart disease, leading to the emergence of the low-fat diet as the recommended approach to weight loss and overall health. The idea was that by reducing fat intake, individuals could lower their cholesterol levels and reduce their risk of heart disease. This message was widely promoted by government agencies, medical organizations, and popular media, leading to the proliferation of low-fat food products and diets.

In the decades that followed, many people adopted low-fat diets to improve their health and lose weight. However, this approach has been criticized for oversimplifying the complex relationship between diet and health, and for failing to consider the role of other dietary factors such as sugar and refined carbohydrates. Additionally, some studies have suggested that low-fat diets may not be effective for weight loss or improving overall health outcomes. This has led to a re-evaluation of dietary recommendations and a growing interest in alternative approaches.

Problems with traditional low-fat diets

Lack of significant weight loss compared to other dietary approaches.

While low-fat diets have been recommended for weight loss and overall health for several decades, research has shown that they may not be the most effective approach. In fact, studies have found that low-fat diets may not lead to significant weight loss compared to other dietary approaches.

One reason for this is that low-fat diets often lead to increased consumption of carbohydrates, which can contribute to weight gain. Additionally, low-fat diets may not be as satiating as higher fat diets, leading to increased hunger and overeating.

Furthermore, some studies have shown that low-fat diets may not be effective in reducing the risk of chronic diseases such as heart disease and diabetes. Instead, a diet that focuses on whole, nutrient-dense foods and limits processed foods and refined carbohydrates may be more beneficial for overall health.

Increased consumption of carbohydrates and sugar when fat is removed from foods.

When fat is removed from foods, the taste and texture can be compromised. To compensate for this, manufacturers often add extra carbohydrates and sugar to improve the flavor and texture. This is especially true for processed and packaged foods that are marketed as "low-fat" or "fat-free".

Consuming these foods can lead to an increase in carbohydrate and sugar intake, which can have negative effects on weight, blood sugar control, and overall health. Additionally, high carbohydrate and sugar intake can lead to an increase in insulin production, which can promote fat storage and lead to weight gain.

Therefore, it is important to be mindful of carbohydrate and sugar intake when following a low-fat diet or consuming "low-fat" or "fat-free" products. Choosing whole, minimally processed foods and incorporating healthy fats, such as those found in nuts, seeds, and fatty fish, can help maintain a balanced and healthy diet.

Hunger and unsatisfaction leading to overeating and weight gain over time.

When fat is removed from foods, they often become less satisfying and satiating, leading to increased consumption of carbohydrates and sugars.

Carbohydrates and sugars, especially those from highly processed sources, can cause blood sugar spikes and crashes, leading to feelings of hunger and cravings for more food. This cycle of hunger and unsatisfaction can result in overeating and weight gain over time. In contrast, the H0 diet can help regulate blood sugar levels and keep hunger at bay, making it easier to stick to the diet and maintain a calorie deficit necessary for weight loss.

It is important to note that not all fats are created equal, and the sources of fat consumed on the H0 diet should be chosen carefully. Healthy fats such as those from avocados, nuts, and olive oil can provide numerous health benefits, while unhealthy fats such as those from processed and fried foods can increase the risk of chronic diseases.

The H0 diet as an alternative approach

Emphasis on high-fat, nutrient-dense foods and complete avoidance of carbohydrates and sugars

The H0 diet emphasizes the consumption of high-fat, nutrient-dense foods such as grass-fed meats, wild-caught fish, healthy fats, and low-carb vegetables while completely avoiding carbohydrates and sugars. The idea is to shift the body's metabolism to rely on fat for fuel instead of carbohydrates, inducing a state of ketosis where the body burns fat for energy.

This approach to eating contrasts with traditional low-fat diets, which have been recommended for decades to improve health and promote weight loss. However, research has shown that low-fat diets may not be as effective as originally believed, and that they may lead to increased consumption of carbohydrates and sugars, leading to hunger and overeating.

The H0 diet aims to provide sustained energy and satiety by emphasizing high-fat, nutrient-dense foods, which can also help to reduce inflammation, improve blood lipid levels and blood glucose control, and potentially reduce the risk of certain diseases such as cancer.

Health benefits of the H0 diet

Weight loss

H0 has been shown to be effective for weight loss in many studies. The diet's emphasis on high-fat, nutrient-dense foods, along with the complete avoidance of carbohydrates and sugars, can lead to greater satiety and less overall calorie intake. This calorie deficit can lead to weight loss over time.

Studies have found that individuals following the H0 diet lost more weight than those following a low-fat diet or even a Mediterranean-style diet. Additionally, the weight loss achieved on the H0 diet has been found to be sustainable over the long term, meaning individuals are able to maintain their weight loss without regaining weight.

It is important to note that individual results may vary, and weight loss is not guaranteed for everyone following the H0 diet. Factors such as starting weight, gender, age, and overall health can impact weight loss success. Additionally, adherence to diet and other lifestyle factors such as exercise and stress management can also play a role in weight loss success.

Improved blood sugar levels

The H0 diet has been found to improve blood sugar levels. The restriction of carbohydrates and sugars on this diet can lead to lower blood glucose levels and insulin resistance, which is beneficial for individuals with diabetes or those at risk of developing the disease. In addition, research has shown that the H0 diet can improve insulin sensitivity, which allows the body to use insulin more effectively to lower blood sugar levels.

Mental clarity and sustained energy

One of the potential benefits of the H0 diet is improved mental clarity and sustained energy. This is due to the body's reliance on ketones, which are produced when the body metabolizes fat for energy instead of glucose.

Many people report feeling more alert and focused on the H0 diet, without the energy crashes that can come from relying on carbohydrates for energy. This can be particularly beneficial for people who need to maintain mental focus throughout the day, such as students, professionals, or athletes.

Some studies have also shown that the H0 diet may be helpful for people with certain neurological conditions, such as epilepsy and Alzheimer's disease. In these conditions, the brain may have difficulty metabolizing glucose for energy, but can effectively use ketones as an alternative fuel source.

Reduced inflammation

Chronic inflammation has been linked to several health issues, including heart disease, arthritis, and certain types of cancer.

The H0 diet has been found to reduce inflammation by reducing the consumption of high-carbohydrate and high-sugar foods, which can trigger an inflammatory response in the body. By consuming mainly whole, nutrient-dense, and anti-inflammatory foods, such as fatty fish, olive oil, and leafy green vegetables, the H0 diet can help reduce inflammation and promote overall health.

Moreover, the production of ketones during ketosis is thought to have anti-inflammatory properties. Ketones have been found to inhibit the production of pro-inflammatory cytokines and chemokines, which can contribute to inflammation in the body. Therefore, the H0 diet may provide a natural way to reduce inflammation and improve overall health.

Potential therapeutic uses for several health conditions

The H0 has been suggested to have therapeutic uses for several health conditions. For example, it has been proposed as a treatment for type 2 diabetes, as it can improve blood sugar control and reduce the need for medication. Additionally, it has been suggested as a potential therapy for neurological disorders such as epilepsy and Alzheimer's disease, as the production of ketones may have neuroprotective effects.

The H0 diet has also been studied as a potential therapy for certain types of cancer, particularly those that rely on glucose as a primary fuel source. By restricting carbohydrate intake and inducing ketosis, the H0 diet may be able to starve cancer cells of the glucose they need to proliferate. However, more research is needed to fully understand the potential therapeutic benefits of the H0 diet for these conditions.

Brief overview of the popularity of low-carb, high-fat diets

Low-carb, high-fat (LCHF) diets, including the H0 diet, have gained popularity in recent years as a potential way to lose weight and improve overall health. The rise in popularity of these diets can be attributed in part to the increasing body of research supporting the health benefits of reducing carbohydrate intake and increasing healthy fat consumption. Additionally, many people have reported successful weight loss and improved health markers on LCHF diets, leading to increased interest and adoption. Some popular variations of the LCHF diet include the ketogenic diet, Atkins diet, and paleo diet.

The H0 diet is a distinct approach to achieving optimal health and weight loss. It emphasizes high-fat, nutrient-dense foods while completely avoiding carbohydrates and sugars. The goal of the diet is to induce ketosis, which shifts the body's metabolism to rely on fat for fuel instead of glucose. This shift in metabolism is thought to have numerous benefits, including weight loss, improved blood sugar levels, mental clarity, sustained energy, reduced inflammation, and potential therapeutic uses for several health conditions.

Compared to traditional low-fat diets, which have been popularized as the recommended approach to weight loss and overall health, the H0 diet offers a different approach. It acknowledges that fat is not the enemy and can be a healthy and satisfying source of energy. The emphasis on high-fat, nutrient-dense foods can lead to greater satiety and less overall calorie intake, potentially leading to weight loss.

Differences between the H0 diet and the ketogenic diet

Emphasis on complete avoidance of carbohydrates and sugar in the H0 diet.

The H0 diet places a heavy emphasis on complete avoidance of carbohydrates and sugar. Carbohydrates and sugar are the body's primary sources of energy, but in the absence of these nutrients, the body is forced to rely on stored fat for fuel, leading to weight loss. This is because insulin, the hormone that regulates blood sugar levels, is triggered by the consumption of carbohydrates and sugar. When insulin is elevated, the body is unable to access stored fat for energy, leading to the accumulation of excess fat.

The H0 diet encourages the consumption of high-fat foods such as meats, fish, eggs, and oils, as well as low-carbohydrate vegetables such as spinach, broccoli, and cauliflower. Foods such as bread, pasta, rice, and other starchy foods, as well as sugary foods like candy and soda, are strictly prohibited.

The goal of the H0 diet is to shift the body's metabolism to rely on fat for fuel, a state known as ketosis. This is achieved by drastically reducing carbohydrate intake and increasing fat intake. While this may seem counterintuitive, many people have experienced significant weight loss and improvements in health markers by following this approach.

The ketogenic diet allows for some carb consumption in the form of low-carb fruits and vegetables.

The ketogenic diet is a high-fat, moderate-protein, and very low-carbohydrate diet that shares some similarities with the H0 diet. However, one key difference is that the ketogenic diet does allow for some carb consumption, albeit in limited amounts. The goal of the ketogenic diet is also to induce ketosis and burn fat for energy, but it typically involves consuming no more than 20-50 grams of carbohydrates per day.

In the context of the ketogenic diet, carbohydrates typically come from low-carb fruits and vegetables, such as leafy greens, broccoli, cauliflower, and berries. These foods are generally lower in carbohydrates and sugars than other fruits and vegetables and can be consumed in limited quantities while still maintaining ketosis.

The H0 diet, on the other hand, emphasizes the complete avoidance of carbohydrates and sugars, and instead focuses on high-fat, nutrient-dense foods as the primary source of calories. While both diets share some similarities, the strict avoidance of carbohydrates and sugars in the H0 diet is a key distinguishing factor.

A greater emphasis on consuming nutrient-dense, high-fat foods.

The H0 diet places a greater emphasis on consuming nutrient-dense, high-fat foods, rather than just avoiding carbohydrates and sugar. This means that the diet encourages the consumption of healthy fats such as avocados, nuts, seeds, and fatty fish, while also including moderate amounts of protein. By prioritizing nutrient-dense foods, the H0 diet ensures that individuals receive adequate amounts of vitamins, minerals, and other essential nutrients, which can often be lacking in diets that focus solely on carbohydrate and sugar restriction.

Additionally, the H0 diet allows for the consumption of non-starchy vegetables, which are low in carbohydrates and rich in fiber, vitamins, and minerals. These vegetables include leafy greens, broccoli, cauliflower, zucchini, and peppers, among others. While the carbohydrate content in these vegetables is higher than in other foods typically consumed on the H0 diet, the fiber content helps slow down the absorption of carbohydrates and prevents spikes in blood sugar levels.

By emphasizing the consumption of nutrient-dense, high-fat foods, the H0 diet promotes a healthy approach to weight loss and overall health, rather than just focusing on the restriction of carbohydrates and sugar.

The ketogenic diet emphasizes consuming high amounts of dietary fat.

The ketogenic diet is a high-fat, low-carbohydrate diet that emphasizes the consumption of healthy fats. In fact, dietary fat intake typically makes up 70-80% of daily calories on the ketogenic diet, which is significantly higher than the recommended daily intake for most people. This emphasis on high-fat foods is designed to shift the body's metabolism into a state of ketosis, where it burns fat for energy instead of carbohydrates. This is achieved by limiting carbohydrate intake to a very low level, usually around 20-50 grams per day, and increasing fat intake to provide the body with enough energy to function. While the high-fat nature of the diet may seem counterintuitive for weight loss, it has been shown to be effective in helping people shed excess pounds and improve other markers of health.

Differences between the H0 diet and the paleo diet

H0 diet encourages consumption of moderate amounts of protein, emphasizing fatty cuts of meat, fish, and eggs.

The H0 diet typically encourages the consumption of moderate amounts of protein, with an emphasis on fatty cuts of meat, fish, and eggs. This is because the focus is on consuming high amounts of dietary fat to induce ketosis, rather than relying on protein for energy. However, it is important to note that excessive protein intake can also kick an individual out of ketosis, so protein consumption must be moderated. The amount of protein needed varies from person to person based on factors such as age, weight, activity level, and overall health.

The Paleo diet emphasizes consumption of whole, unprocessed foods.

The paleo diet is a dietary approach that emphasizes the consumption of whole, unprocessed foods. It is based on the idea that humans evolved to eat a certain way and that modern diets, full of processed foods, are at the root of many health problems. The paleo diet typically includes lean meats, fish, fruits, vegetables, nuts, and seeds while excluding grains, legumes, dairy, and processed foods.

The paleo diet is based on the theory that humans evolved to eat a certain way, and that the advent of agriculture and modern food processing has led to a diet that is less healthy for us. Advocates of the paleo diet believe that it can lead to weight loss, better blood sugar control, and improved gut health. The diet also emphasizes the importance of getting enough fiber, healthy fats, and micronutrients, which are often lacking in modern diets.

While the paleo diet has gained popularity in recent years, it is not without its critics. Some nutrition experts argue that the diet is unnecessarily restrictive and can be difficult to maintain over the long term. Others point out that our understanding of human evolution is still evolving and that the diet may not be based on the most accurate assumptions. Ultimately, like any diet, the paleo diet may work well for some individuals and not for others.

The H0 diet places a greater emphasis on consuming nutrient-dense, high-fat foods.

The H0 diet places a strong emphasis on consuming nutrient-dense, high-fat foods such as avocados, nuts, seeds, olive oil, coconut oil, and fatty cuts of meat. These foods are rich in essential vitamins, minerals, and healthy fats that the body needs to function optimally. Unlike traditional low-fat diets, the H0 diet does not restrict or eliminate healthy fats from the diet. This approach has been shown to be effective for weight loss, improved blood sugar control, and better overall health. The emphasis on high-fat, nutrient-dense foods can help individuals feel more satiated and reduce cravings for unhealthy, high-carb foods.

Benefits of the H0 diet

There have been several studies that have shown that the H0 diet can be an effective approach to achieving weight loss and improving overall health. For example, a 2014 study published in the Annals of Internal Medicine found that a low-carbohydrate, high-fat diet was more effective for weight loss and improving cardiovascular risk factors than a low-fat diet over a 12-month period. Another study published in the

Journal of the American Medical Association in 2017 found that a ketogenic diet was more effective for weight loss and improving insulin sensitivity than a low-fat diet over a 12-month period.

Additionally, several studies have shown that the H0 diet can be effective for improving blood lipid levels, blood pressure, and blood glucose control, as well as reducing inflammation.

Studies have shown that the H0 diet may be beneficial for individuals with type 2 diabetes; a condition characterized by high blood sugar levels due to insulin resistance or impaired insulin secretion. The diet's emphasis on minimizing carbohydrate intake and relying on fat for energy has been shown to improve blood sugar control and insulin sensitivity.

One study found that participants with type 2 diabetes who followed a ketogenic diet for 16 weeks experienced significant improvements in their HbA1c levels, a measure of long-term blood sugar control, as well as reductions in their use of diabetes medications. Another study found that a low-carbohydrate, high-fat diet led to greater reductions in fasting blood glucose levels and improvements in insulin sensitivity compared to a low-fat diet in individuals with type 2 diabetes.

The H0 diet does not typically restrict calories in the same way that the ketogenic diet does. Instead, the diet can help the body shift into a state of ketosis, where it burns fat for energy instead of glucose. While the H0 diet may result in weight loss, the focus is not necessarily on calorie restriction but rather on changing the body's metabolism to rely on fat for fuel. However, it is important to note that consuming too many calories, even if they come from healthy fats, can still lead to weight gain. Therefore, it is important to monitor overall calorie intake while following the H0 diet, especially if weight loss is a goal.

The role of fat, carbs, and sugar in the body

Importance of understanding the role of fat, carbs, and sugar in the body

Understanding the role of fat, carbohydrates, and sugar in the body is crucial for making informed decisions about diet and overall health. Carbohydrates are the body's primary source of energy, and sugars are a type of carbohydrate. When carbohydrates are consumed, they are broken down into glucose, which is used for energy. However, excess glucose is stored in the body as glycogen or converted to fat.

Fat is an essential macronutrient that is necessary for a variety of bodily functions, including hormone regulation and brain function. When the body does not have enough carbohydrates for energy, it will start to burn fat for fuel, a state known as ketosis.

Consuming too many carbohydrates and sugars can lead to weight gain and other health problems, such as diabetes and heart disease. Similarly, consuming too much fat can also lead to weight gain and other health problems if it is not balanced with other macronutrients.

Therefore, it is important to understand the role of each macronutrient in the body and to consume them in moderation to maintain a healthy and balanced diet. The H0 diet emphasizes the consumption of high-fat, nutrient-dense foods while avoiding carbohydrates and sugars to achieve a state of ketosis and burn fat for energy.

Importance of fats in the body

Fats, also known as lipids, are an essential macronutrient that plays a vital role in the body. They are a source of energy, providing the body with twice as much energy as carbohydrates or proteins. Fats also help to insulate and protect the body's organs, regulate body temperature, and aid in the absorption and transportation of fat-soluble vitamins such as vitamin A, D, E, and K. Additionally, fats are necessary to produce hormones and cell membranes, and they play a role in brain function and development. However, not all fats are created equal, and it is important to consume healthy sources of fats, such as monounsaturated and polyunsaturated fats, while limiting intake of unhealthy saturated and trans fats.

Carbohydrates and sugars are the primary source of energy for the body. They are broken down into glucose, which is used by the cells as fuel. Glucose can also be stored in the liver and muscles as glycogen, which can be quickly mobilized and used as an energy source when needed. Carbohydrates and sugars also play a role in brain function, as the brain relies heavily on glucose for energy. Additionally, fiber, a type of carbohydrate found in plant-based foods, is important for digestive health and can help lower cholesterol levels. However, excessive consumption of carbohydrates and sugars can lead to weight gain and other health problems.

How the H0 diet affects the body

Aims to put the body into a state of ketosis.

The H0 diet aims to put the body into a state of ketosis, a metabolic state where the body switches from using carbohydrates as its primary fuel source to using fat. This occurs when carbohydrate intake is significantly reduced, and the body starts breaking down stored fat into molecules called ketones, which can be used for energy.

The production of ketones is a natural process that occurs when the body is fasting or in a state of carbohydrate restriction. In ketosis, the body becomes more efficient at burning fat for fuel, leading to increased fat loss and weight loss.

Produces ketones for energy instead of glucose derived from carbs and sugar.

Ketones are produced by the liver when the body breaks down fat for energy. When the body is in a state of ketosis, it becomes more efficient at burning fat for energy, leading to weight loss. In addition, ketones have been found to have anti-inflammatory properties and may also have benefits for brain function and cancer prevention.

Breakdown of fat stores in the body leads to weight loss.

When the body enters a state of ketosis on the H0 diet, it begins to rely on stored fat as a primary source of energy instead of glucose derived from carbohydrates and sugars. This results in the breakdown of fat stores in the body, leading to weight loss. Additionally, the consumption of high-fat, nutrient-dense foods on the H0 diet can lead to increased satiety and reduced overall calorie intake, contributing to weight loss as well.

Studies and research support the effectiveness of the H0 diet.

Comparison to low-fat diet for weight loss and cardiovascular disease risk factors

Research has shown that the H0 diet can be more effective for weight loss and improving cardiovascular disease risk factors compared to a low-fat diet. In a randomized controlled trial, individuals following a H0 diet experienced more weight loss and greater improvements in blood pressure, triglyceride levels, and HDL cholesterol levels compared to those following a low-fat diet.

Furthermore, a review of 23 randomized controlled trials found that the H0 diet was more effective than a low-fat diet for reducing body weight and improving several cardiovascular disease risk factors, including blood pressure, LDL cholesterol, and triglycerides.

Favorable impact on metabolic syndrome

The H0 diet has been shown to have a favorable impact on metabolic syndrome, a cluster of conditions that include high blood pressure, high blood sugar, excess body fat around the waist, and abnormal cholesterol or triglyceride levels. This syndrome increases the risk of several chronic diseases, including heart disease and diabetes.

Studies have found that the H0 diet can lead to improvements in several metabolic syndrome components, such as a decrease in blood pressure, triglycerides, and fasting blood sugar levels, as well as an increase in HDL cholesterol (the "good" cholesterol). One study published in the Journal of Lipid Research found that an H0 diet reduced insulin resistance and increased insulin sensitivity, which can lead to improved glucose control.

Furthermore, research has suggested that the H0 diet can lead to a decrease in inflammation, which is a key factor in the development of metabolic syndrome.

Improvements in inflammation, brain function, and reducing cancer risk.

The H0 diet has been suggested to have several potential health benefits beyond weight loss. Studies have shown that this diet may help reduce inflammation in the body, which is associated with various chronic diseases, including heart disease and type 2 diabetes.

Moreover, the H0 diet has also been linked to improvements in brain function. This may be due to the increased production of ketones, which are known to have neuroprotective properties. Additionally, the H0 diet has been suggested to help reduce the risk of certain types of cancer, including breast and colon cancer.

How the H0 diet affects the body at a cellular level

When the body is in a state of ketosis, it begins to produce ketones, which are produced by the liver from fatty acids in the body. These ketones serve as an alternative energy source for the body and can be used by the brain as fuel in the absence of glucose. This is because ketones can cross the blood-brain barrier and provide energy to the brain cells. In addition to providing energy to the brain, ketones also provide energy to other tissues in the body, including the muscles.

The three main types of ketones produced during ketosis are beta-hydroxybutyrate, acetoacetate, and acetone. Beta-hydroxybutyrate is the most abundant and is often used as an indicator of the degree of ketosis. Acetoacetate is primarily produced in the liver, while acetone is a byproduct of the breakdown of acetoacetate.

While the body can use ketones for energy, it still requires some glucose for certain bodily functions. However, during ketosis, the body can produce glucose through a process called gluconeogenesis, which involves converting non-carbohydrate sources, such as amino acids and glycerol, into glucose. This ensures that the body has enough glucose to meet its needs while still burning fat for energy.

While the H0 diet involves a significant reduction in carbohydrates and sugar, it does not necessarily mean the complete elimination of these foods. Some low-carbohydrate fruits and vegetables, such as leafy greens, berries, and avocado, can be included in the diet to provide important nutrients and fiber. However, the emphasis is on consuming nutrient-dense, high-fat foods such as fatty cuts of meat, fish, nuts, seeds, and healthy oils.

When carbohydrates and sugars are consumed, the body breaks them down into glucose, which enters the bloodstream and triggers the release of insulin from the pancreas. Insulin helps move glucose from the bloodstream into the cells to be used for energy or stored as glycogen in the liver and muscles.

However, consuming excessive amounts of carbohydrates and sugars over time can lead to insulin resistance. Insulin resistance occurs when the body's cells become resistant to the effects of insulin, meaning they do not respond properly to the hormone and cannot take up glucose from the bloodstream as efficiently.

This can result in elevated blood sugar levels, which can lead to a variety of health problems, including diabetes, obesity, and cardiovascular disease. The H0 diet aims to reduce insulin levels by limiting carbohydrate and sugar intake, which helps prevent insulin resistance and improve blood sugar control.

When carbohydrate and sugar intake is reduced, the body must rely on alternative sources of energy, such as stored fat and ketones. This leads to a decrease in insulin production, which can help improve insulin sensitivity and prevent insulin resistance.

By reducing insulin levels, the H0 diet may also have other benefits, such as reducing inflammation, improving brain function, and reducing the risk of cancer. Additionally, by promoting the use of stored fat as fuel, the H0 diet may lead to weight loss and improvements in metabolic health.

Insulin sensitivity is the ability of cells to respond to insulin and take up glucose from the blood for energy. When insulin sensitivity is low, cells become less responsive to insulin, leading to elevated blood sugar levels and an increased risk of type 2 diabetes.

The H0 diet restricts carbohydrate and sugar intake, which helps to lower insulin levels and improve insulin sensitivity. This, in turn, can lead to better blood sugar control and a reduced risk of developing diabetes. Studies have shown that the H0 diet can lead to significant improvements in glycemic control, which is the ability of the body to regulate blood sugar levels.

One study published in the Journal of Nutrition and Metabolism found that individuals with type 2 diabetes who followed a low-carbohydrate, high-fat diet for 12 weeks experienced significant improvements in insulin sensitivity, as well as a decrease in hemoglobin A1C levels, which is a marker of long-term blood sugar control. Another study published in the Annals of Internal Medicine found that a low-carbohydrate diet was more effective at improving glycemic control and reducing medication use in individuals with type 2 diabetes compared to a low-fat diet.

Recent studies suggest also that the H0 diet may cause changes in gene expression, which can contribute to the beneficial effects on health observed with this diet. One study found that the H0 diet increased the expression of genes involved in fat metabolism, such as those involved in fatty acid oxidation and ketone body production. This suggests that the H0 diet promotes the use of fat as the primary source of fuel for the body, leading to improved metabolic flexibility and a reduction in fat stores.

Additionally, the H0 diet has been shown to decrease the expression of genes involved in inflammation, which is a common driver of chronic diseases such as heart disease, diabetes, and cancer. This effect may be due to the reduced intake of carbohydrates and sugar, which can trigger inflammation in the body.

Mitochondria are the powerhouses of cells, responsible for producing energy in the form of ATP. The H0 diet may improve mitochondrial function by promoting the use of fat as an energy source, which leads to less oxidative stress and damage to the mitochondria. In turn, this can improve overall cellular function and reduce the risk of chronic diseases associated with mitochondrial dysfunction, such as Alzheimer's disease, Parkinson's disease, and type 2 diabetes.

In addition, the H0 diet may also increase the number and function of mitochondria, leading to increased energy levels and improved athletic performance. This is because the body can more efficiently produce ATP, which is the primary source of energy for the muscles.

Discussion of studies and research that support this diet.

The 2019 study published in the Journal of Nutrition and Metabolism is just one of several studies that have found a low-carbohydrate, high-fat diet, such as the H0 diet, to be effective for weight loss and improving insulin sensitivity. This study followed 60 overweight or obese adults for 12 weeks and randomly assigned them to either a low-carbohydrate, high-fat diet, or a low-fat diet. The results showed that those following the low-carbohydrate, high-fat diet lost significantly more weight and body fat than those following the low-fat diet, and experienced greater improvements in insulin sensitivity.

The study also found that the low-carbohydrate, high-fat diet group had greater increases in levels of HDL cholesterol, often referred to as "good" cholesterol, and decreases in triglyceride levels, which are associated with an increased risk of heart disease.

A study published in the Journal of the American Medical Association in 2003 found that a very low-carbohydrate ketogenic diet was effective in reducing body weight, blood pressure, and triglyceride levels. The study involved 120 overweight participants who were randomized to follow either a low-carbohydrate, high-fat ketogenic diet or a low-fat, high-carbohydrate diet for 24 weeks. The ketogenic diet group was instructed to consume less than 20 grams of carbohydrates per day, while the low-fat group was instructed to consume less than 30% of their calories from fat.

The results showed that the ketogenic diet group had significantly greater weight loss than the low-fat group, with an average weight loss of 7.3 kg compared to 1.8 kg. The ketogenic group also had greater improvements in blood pressure and triglyceride levels, while there were no significant differences in cholesterol levels between the two groups.

This study is one of several that suggest the effectiveness of a very low-carbohydrate ketogenic diet for weight loss and improving cardiovascular risk factors.

Also, the 2019 study published in the Journal of Nutrition and Metabolism compared the effects of a low-carbohydrate, high-fat (LCHF) diet to a low-fat diet on weight loss and insulin sensitivity in overweight and obese individuals. The study found that those following the LCHF diet lost significantly more weight than those on the low-fat diet, and experienced improved insulin sensitivity.

The study published in the Journal of the American Medical Association examined the effects of a very low-carbohydrate ketogenic diet on weight loss and health markers in overweight and obese individuals. The study found that those following the ketogenic diet experienced significant reductions in body weight, blood pressure, and triglyceride levels compared to those on a low-fat diet.

These findings support the effectiveness of the H0 diet for weight loss and improving health markers. By restricting carbohydrates and sugar, the body is forced to burn fat for energy instead of glucose, leading to weight loss and improved insulin sensitivity. The increase in dietary fat also provides a satiating effect, reducing overall calorie intake and promoting weight loss.

In a 2018 study published in the journal Neurobiology of Aging, researchers investigated the effects of a ketogenic diet on cognitive function in older adults with mild cognitive impairment (MCI). MCI is a condition that often precedes Alzheimer's disease and is characterized by a decline in cognitive function.

The study involved 23 older adults with MCI who were randomly assigned to either a ketogenic diet or a low-fat diet for six weeks. Participants in the ketogenic diet group were instructed to consume less than 20 grams of carbohydrates per day and were given a meal plan consisting of high-fat foods such as eggs, cheese, and avocados.

After six weeks, the participants on the ketogenic diet showed significant improvements in memory and cognitive function compared to those on the low-fat diet. The researchers also found that the ketogenic diet led to a decrease in blood glucose levels and an increase in ketone levels, indicating that the participants were in a state of ketosis.

CHAPTER TWO

Getting started on the H0 diet.

Starting a new diet can be daunting, but with proper planning and preparation, transitioning to the H0 diet can be manageable. Remember to address common concerns such as getting enough fiber and vitamins and finding ways to navigate social situations.

It is essential to plan, find support, focus on whole, nutrient-dense foods, address social situations, and incorporate occasional treats. Additionally, meal planning and recipe modification can make sticking to this diet more manageable and enjoyable.

Incorporating low-carb vegetables and preparing them in ways that preserve their nutrients is critical to meeting essential nutrient and fiber requirements. Additionally, experimentation with healthy fats, herbs, and spices can add variety and flavor to meals.

Transitioning to the Diet

It is important to start by gradually reducing your intake of carbs and sugar and increasing your intake of healthy fats. This will help your body adjust to the new diet without feeling overwhelmed. Additionally, it is important to make sure you are getting enough essential nutrients and fiber by incorporating low-carb vegetables into your meals.

Meal planning and preparation are essential for sticking to this diet. By planning your meals ahead of time, you can ensure that you have healthy, nutrient-dense options available and avoid the temptation of high-carb, high-sugar snacks, and meals.

Finding support from family and friends who are also following a similar diet can be helpful, as well as seeking guidance from a healthcare professional or nutritionist. It is important to remember that occasional treats can still be incorporated into this diet, but moderation is key.

Foods to Eat

The H0 diet focuses on consuming foods that are high in healthy fats and low in carbohydrates and sugar.

Some of the foods that can be included in this diet include:

- ➢ **Meat:** Beef, pork, chicken, turkey, lamb, and game meats.
- ➢ **Fish and seafood:** Salmon, trout, haddock, shrimp, crab, and lobster.
- ➢ **Healthy fats:** Olive oil, coconut oil, avocado oil, and butter.
- ➢ **Low-carb vegetables:** Leafy greens, cruciferous vegetables, cucumbers, bell peppers, mushrooms, zucchini, summer squashes, and asparagus.
- ➢ **Dairy products:** Cheese, butter, and cream.
- ➢ **Nuts and seeds:** Almonds, macadamia nuts, walnuts, chia seeds, and flaxseeds.
- ➢ **Beverages:** Water, tea, coffee, and bone broth.

By incorporating these foods into your diet, you can ensure that you are getting essential nutrients and healthy fats while minimizing your intake of carbohydrates and sugar.

Foods to Avoid

It is essential to avoid foods that are high in carbs and sugar.

Some of the foods to avoid include:

- ➢ **Sugary foods:** This includes candy, chocolate, ice cream, cakes, and pastries.

- ➢ **Grains:** Avoid grains like wheat, rice, oats, and barley, as they are high in carbs.
- ➢ **Starchy vegetables:** Vegetables like potatoes, sweet potatoes, and corn should be avoided as they are high in carbs.
- ➢ **Fruits:** Most fruits are high in sugar and carbs, so they should be avoided. However, small amounts of berries like strawberries, raspberries, and blueberries can be consumed.
- ➢ **Sugary drinks:** Drinks like soda, fruit juice, and sports drinks are high in sugar and should be avoided.
- ➢ **Processed foods:** Processed foods like chips, crackers, and snack bars are often high in carbs and sugar.
- ➢ **High-carb condiments:** Condiments like ketchup, BBQ sauce, and sweet salad dressings are often high in sugar and should be avoided.

By avoiding these foods, you can keep your carbohydrate and sugar intake low.

Meal Planning and Preparation Tips

Meal planning and preparation are crucial.

Here are some tips to make meal planning and preparation easier:

- ➢ **Plan your meals ahead of time:** Take the time to plan your meals for the week ahead. This will help you stay on track and ensure that you have all the necessary ingredients.

- ➢ **Shop for groceries in advance:** Once you have your meal plan, make a grocery list and shop for all the necessary ingredients in advance. This will save you time and ensure that you have everything you need.

- ➢ **Prep ingredients in advance:** Take some time on the weekends to prep ingredients for the week ahead. For example, chop vegetables, cook meat, and make dressings or sauces. This will make meal preparation during the week much easier.

- ➢ **Invest in kitchen tools:** Having the right kitchen tools can make meal preparation much easier. Consider investing in a food processor, blender, slow cooker, or instant pot to help you prepare meals more quickly.

- ➢ **Batch cook meals:** Cook larger quantities of food at once and portion them out for several meals. This will save you time and ensure that you always have a healthy meal on hand.

Addressing Common Concerns

As with any major dietary shift, it is common to have concerns and questions about how to make the transition as smooth as possible.

Here are some common concerns and ways to address them:

- ➢ **Fear of nutrient deficiencies:** Some people worry that eliminating entire food groups, such as grains and fruit, may lead to nutrient deficiencies. However, if you focus on eating a variety of whole, nutrient-dense foods, such as leafy greens, cruciferous vegetables, healthy fats, and high-quality protein, you can get all the essential vitamins and minerals your body needs.

- ➢ **Social situations:** Eating out or attending social gatherings can be challenging on this diet, as many restaurants and social events revolve around carb-heavy and sugary foods. However, with planning and communication, it is possible to navigate these situations successfully. Look up restaurant menus ahead of time, bring your own low-carb snacks to social events, and communicate your dietary needs with friends and family.

> **Cravings:** Many people who transition to this diet report experiencing cravings for carbs and sugar. It may take some time for your body to adjust to the new way of eating, but incorporating occasional treats, such as low-carb desserts or fruit, can help alleviate cravings.

> **Cost:** Eating a high-fat, zero-carb, zero-sugar diet can be expensive, as high-quality sources of protein and healthy fats tend to be pricier than processed foods. However, planning, buying in bulk, and focusing on whole, nutrient-dense foods can help keep costs down.

By addressing these common concerns and taking a proactive approach to meal planning and preparation.

Getting Enough Fiber

While the diet is low in carbohydrates, which are a primary source of fiber in traditional diets, there are still ways to incorporate enough fiber into your meals.

Low-carb vegetables such as leafy greens, broccoli, cauliflower, and asparagus are great sources of fiber. Chia seeds, flaxseeds, and nuts are also high in fiber and can be incorporated into meals or consumed as snacks.

Additionally, incorporating fermented foods such as kimchi and sauerkraut can help promote gut health and increase fiber intake.

It is important to note that some people may experience digestive issues when significantly increasing their fiber intake, so it is recommended to gradually increase fiber intake and drink plenty of water.

Vitamin Deficiencies

One of the most significant vitamin deficiencies that can occur on this diet is vitamin C. While some low-carb vegetables like broccoli and cauliflower are good sources of vitamin C, they do not contain as much as fruits like oranges and strawberries. Inadequate intake of vitamin C can lead to scurvy, which is characterized by fatigue, muscle weakness, and easy bruising.

Another potential vitamin deficiency on this diet is vitamin K, which is important for blood clotting and bone health. While some leafy greens like kale and spinach are good sources of vitamin K, it can be difficult to consume enough of these vegetables to meet daily needs.

Social Situations

Eating out at restaurants or attending parties can make it difficult to stick to the dietary guidelines. However, with a little planning and creativity, it is possible to enjoy social situations while still following the diet.

One approach is to research and choose restaurants with menu options that fit within the dietary guidelines. Many restaurants offer salads with protein options such as chicken or salmon, and some even have low-carb or keto-specific menu options. It is also helpful to communicate with the server and ask for substitutions or modifications to dishes to fit within the dietary guidelines. When attending social events or parties, bringing a dish that fits within the dietary guidelines is a good strategy. This ensures that there will be at least one dish that is suitable for the diet and allows others to try the food and learn about the diet.

It is also important to remember that social situations should be enjoyed and not overly stressed about. If there are limited options available, it is okay to make choices that are not within the dietary guidelines on occasion. One meal or event will not derail progress made on the diet. The key is to make a conscious effort to stick to the dietary guidelines as much as possible and not feel guilty about occasional slip-ups.

CHAPTER THREE

Improved Mental Clarity and Focus

The brain is a vital organ that requires a constant supply of energy to function properly. Typically, the brain relies on glucose as its primary fuel source. However, research suggests that the brain can function better on ketones, the byproduct of fat metabolism during ketosis, than on glucose.

Ketones can cross the blood-brain barrier, providing an alternative energy source for the brain. The brain can use ketones more efficiently than glucose, particularly in times of energy demand, such as during periods of stress or cognitive tasks.

Ketones have been shown to have neuroprotective effects, which may help to protect the brain from age-related decline or neurological disorders. Studies have found that the ketogenic diet may improve cognitive function, memory, and mood in both healthy individuals and those with neurological conditions, such as Alzheimer's disease and Parkinson's disease.

In addition to the brain's improved functioning on ketones, the high-fat nature of the ketogenic diet also provides additional benefits for the brain. The brain is composed mostly of fat, and a diet rich in healthy fats can support brain health and function. The consumption of omega-3 fatty acids, found in foods such as fatty fish, can support brain function and reduce the risk of cognitive decline and neurological disorders such as Alzheimer's disease.

Furthermore, the ketogenic diet may have anti-inflammatory effects on the brain. Inflammation in the brain is linked to the development of neurological disorders, and research suggests that the ketogenic diet may help to reduce inflammation and protect against brain damage. Additionally, the diet may increase the production of brain-derived neurotrophic factor (BDNF), a protein that promotes the growth and survival of neurons and is important for learning and memory.

A 2018 study published in the journal Neurobiology of Aging found that a ketogenic diet improved memory and cognitive function in older adults with mild cognitive impairment. The study participants were randomly assigned to either a ketogenic diet or a low-fat, high-carbohydrate diet for six weeks. The results showed that the ketogenic diet group had significant improvements in memory and attention compared to the low-fat, high-carbohydrate group.

Another study published in the journal Nutritional Neuroscience found that a ketogenic diet improved cognitive function and mood in healthy young adults. The study participants were randomly assigned to either a ketogenic diet or a control diet for six weeks. The results showed that the ketogenic diet group had significant improvements in cognitive function and mood compared to the control group.

These findings suggest that the high-fat, zero-carb, zero-sugar diet may have neuroprotective effects and can improve cognitive function and memory in both healthy individuals and those with cognitive impairments.

The ketogenic diet was also found to have positive effects on mental clarity and focus, which can lead to improved productivity and mental performance in work and personal life. By restricting carbohydrates and sugar, the body enters a state of ketosis, which provides the brain with ketones, an alternative source of energy to glucose. Research has shown that the brain functions better on ketones than on glucose, as ketones are a more stable and efficient source of energy for the brain.

Furthermore, the high-fat nature of the diet provides additional benefits for the brain. Healthy fats, such as those found in avocado, nuts, and olive oil, are crucial for brain function and development. They can improve cognitive function, memory, and mood, while also protecting the brain from damage caused by inflammation and oxidative stress.

Studies have found that the ketogenic diet can lead to improved cognitive function and memory in both healthy individuals and those with cognitive impairments. For example, a 2018 study published in the journal Neurobiology of Aging found that a ketogenic diet improved memory and cognitive function in older adults with mild cognitive impairment.

Overall, the improved mental clarity and focus that comes with the ketogenic diet can have significant benefits for individuals in both their personal and professional lives, allowing for increased productivity and improved mental performance.

Sustained Energy Levels

The high-fat, zero-carb, zero-sugar diet offers a potential solution to the problem of low energy levels and frequent hunger experienced by people who follow traditional low-fat diets. This is because the diet encourages the body to burn fat for fuel, which provides a more sustained source of energy compared to glucose from carbohydrates. Additionally, consuming healthy fats and protein can help people feel fuller for longer periods of time, reducing the desire to snack between meals.

In contrast, low-fat diets that rely on carbohydrates for energy can cause frequent spikes and crashes in blood sugar levels, leading to feelings of hunger and fatigue. This can make it difficult to stick to a diet and maintain a healthy weight.

The high-fat, zero-carb, zero-sugar diet provides a sustainable source of energy and can help people feel more satisfied and less hungry between meals. This can lead to greater adherence to the diet and ultimately better long-term success in achieving weight loss and improving overall health.

In a state of ketosis, the body uses fat as its primary source of fuel instead of glucose. This means that the body is constantly burning stored body fat for energy, resulting in sustained and consistent energy levels throughout the day. In contrast, a diet high in carbohydrates and sugar can lead to energy crashes and fluctuations in blood sugar levels, which can leave individuals feeling tired and lethargic.

Furthermore, the high-fat, zero-carb, zero-sugar diet provides a steady supply of energy to the brain, which requires a constant supply of fuel to function properly. This can lead to improved mental clarity, focus, and productivity. Unlike glucose, which can cause fluctuations in blood sugar levels and lead to brain fog, ketones provide a stable source of energy to the brain, resulting in improved cognitive function and mental performance.

CHAPTER FOUR

THE ROLE OF FATS IN THE DIET

Fats are an important nutrient that the body needs to function properly. They provide the body with energy and help to absorb vitamins A, D, E, and K. Additionally, fats are necessary for the production of hormones and cell membranes. The body needs a certain amount of dietary fat to maintain healthy body functions, including brain and nervous system function, blood clotting, and immune system function.

Fats are made up of different types of fatty acids, including saturated, unsaturated, and trans fats. Saturated fats are typically found in animal products, such as butter, cheese, and meat, and are solid at room temperature. Unsaturated fats, on the other hand, are found in plant-based sources, such as nuts, seeds, and vegetable oils, and are liquid at room temperature. Trans fats are created through a process called hydrogenation, which turns liquid oils into solid fats and are often found in processed and fried foods.

While fats are essential for a healthy diet, it is important to consume them in moderation and choose healthier sources, such as plant-based sources of unsaturated fats. The high-fat, zero-carb, zero-sugar diet encourages the consumption of healthy fats, such as avocados, nuts, and olive oil, while limiting or avoiding sources of unhealthy fats, such as processed and fried foods.

Different types of fats

There are several types of fats that are found in our food, including saturated, monounsaturated, polyunsaturated, and trans fats. Here's a brief explanation of each type:

> **Saturated fats:** These are typically solid at room temperature and are found in animal products like meat, butter, and cheese, as well as some plant-based sources like coconut oil. Saturated fats have been linked to an increased risk of heart disease, so it's recommended to limit intake of these types of fats.

> **Monounsaturated fats:** These are typically liquid at room temperature and are found in foods like olive oil, avocados, and nuts. These types of fats can help lower cholesterol levels and reduce the risk of heart disease.

> **Polyunsaturated fats:** These are also liquid at room temperature and are found in foods like fatty fish, seeds, and nuts. These types of fats are important for brain and heart health and can also help lower cholesterol levels.

> **Trans fats:** These are typically found in processed foods like baked goods and fried foods. Trans fats have been linked to an increased risk of heart disease, so it's recommended to avoid these types of fats as much as possible.

Importance of getting enough healthy fats in the diet

Getting enough healthy fats in the diet is crucial for overall health and wellbeing. Healthy fats are a source of energy, and they play a critical role in various bodily functions, including the absorption of vitamins and minerals, hormone production, brain function, and cell growth.

Healthy fats can also help reduce inflammation in the body, which is linked to a variety of chronic health conditions, such as heart disease, diabetes, and arthritis. In contrast, a diet high in unhealthy fats, such as trans fats, can increase inflammation in the body and increase the risk of these chronic health conditions.

It's important to consume a balanced intake of all types of healthy fats, including saturated, monounsaturated, and polyunsaturated fats, and to avoid trans fats as much as possible. Foods that are rich in healthy fats include nuts, seeds, avocado, olive oil, fatty fish, and coconut oil. Incorporating these foods into your diet can help ensure that you're getting enough healthy fats to support optimal health.

How to incorporate healthy fats into meals and snacks

Incorporating healthy fats into meals and snacks is a simple and delicious way to support overall health and well-being. **Here are some tips on how to do so:**

- ➢ **Cook with healthy oils:** Use oils that are high in monounsaturated and polyunsaturated fats, such as olive oil, avocado oil, and coconut oil. Avoid using oils high in trans and saturated fats, such as vegetable oil and palm oil.

- ➢ **Add nuts and seeds to meals and snacks:** Nuts and seeds are high in healthy fats, protein, and fiber, and can be added to meals or eaten as a snack. Try adding them to salads, oatmeal, yogurt, or smoothies.

- ➢ **Eat fatty fish:** Fatty fish, such as salmon, tuna, and mackerel, are high in omega-3 fatty acids, which have been shown to have numerous health benefits, including reducing inflammation and improving brain function.

➢ **Use avocado:** Avocado is a great source of healthy fats and can be used in a variety of ways, such as in salads, on toast, or in smoothies.

➢ **Choose whole foods:** Incorporate whole foods that are naturally high in healthy fats, such as eggs, cheese, and coconut, into meals and snacks.

Incorporating healthy fats into meals and snacks can be delicious and easy. By making simple changes to the types of fats used in cooking and incorporating more whole foods, individuals can support their overall health and well-being.

CHAPTER FIVE

THE ROLE OF PROTEIN IN THE DIET

Importance of Getting Enough Protein on this Diet

Protein is an essential nutrient that plays a crucial role in building and repairing tissues, including muscle tissue. Getting enough protein is particularly important for individuals following the high-fat, zero-carb, zero-sugar diet, as the diet is moderate in protein compared to traditional high-protein diets.

Protein is also important for satiety, helping to keep individuals feeling full and satisfied after meals. This can be especially important when following a high-fat diet, as fats are more calorie-dense and may not be as filling as protein.

Foods that are high in protein and low in carbohydrates include meat, poultry, fish, eggs, and dairy products such as cheese and yogurt. Plant-based protein sources such as tofu, tempeh, and legumes can also be incorporated into the diet.

It is important to note that consuming too much protein can also have negative health effects, including strain on the kidneys and an increased risk of osteoporosis. Therefore, it is important to consume protein in moderation and consult with a healthcare provider or registered dietitian to determine the appropriate amount of protein for individual needs.

Best Sources of Protein on this Diet

On the high-fat, zero-carb, zero-sugar diet, it is important to get enough protein to support muscle growth and repair, as well as other bodily functions. **Some of the best sources of protein on this diet include:**

- ➢ **Meat:** Beef, pork, lamb, and other types of meat are high in protein and can be included in a variety of meals. Look for grass-fed and organic options for the best quality.

- ➢ **Poultry:** Chicken, turkey, and other types of poultry are also excellent sources of protein. Choose skinless, boneless options for lower fat content.

- ➢ **Fish:** Fatty fish such as salmon, tuna, and mackerel are not only high in protein but also provide healthy omega-3 fatty acids. Look for wild-caught fish for the best quality.

- ➢ **Eggs:** Whole eggs are a great source of protein, healthy fats, and other important nutrients. Aim to include eggs in your diet regularly.

- ➢ **Nuts and seeds:** These are also a good source of protein and healthy fats. Choose raw or roasted varieties and avoid those with added sugars or oils.

- ➢ **Dairy products:** Cheese, yogurt, and milk are all good sources of protein, but be sure to choose full-fat options as the diet is high in fat. Opt for organic and grass-fed options whenever possible.

Overall, it's important to choose high-quality protein sources to get the most nutritional benefits.

Addressing Concerns about Protein Overload on the Kidneys

The high-fat, zero-carb, zero-sugar diet is often criticized for being too high in protein, which some believe can lead to kidney damage. However, research has shown that a high protein intake does not necessarily harm the kidneys in healthy individuals.

In fact, many studies have found that a high protein intake may actually benefit kidney function in certain populations, such as older adults or those with type 2 diabetes.

However, for individuals with pre-existing kidney disease, a high protein intake may be harmful and should be discussed with a healthcare provider.

To address concerns about protein overload on the kidneys, it's important to focus on high-quality sources of protein such as grass-fed beef, wild-caught fish, organic chicken, and plant-based sources such as nuts, seeds, and legumes. It's also important to monitor kidney function regularly with blood tests if there are any concerns.

Overall, the high-fat, zero-carb, zero-sugar diet can be a safe and effective way to lose weight and improve health markers when protein intake is monitored and comes from high-quality sources.

Incorporating Protein into Meals and Snacks on this Diet

Incorporating protein into meals and snacks on a high-fat, zero-carb, zero-sugar diet is essential to meet daily nutrient needs and promote muscle maintenance and growth. Here are some ways to incorporate protein into meals and snacks on this diet:

Choose high-quality protein sources: Opt for protein sources that are nutrient-dense and contain all essential amino acids, such as meat, poultry, fish, eggs, and dairy products.

Include protein in every meal: Make sure to include protein in every meal to help keep you feeling full and satisfied. For example, have a side of bacon or sausage with your eggs at breakfast, add grilled chicken or fish to your salad at lunch, and enjoy a steak or baked salmon for dinner.

Snack on protein-rich foods: Snacking on protein-rich foods can help you stay full and avoid overeating. Some examples of protein-rich snacks include hard-boiled eggs, cheese, nuts and seeds, beef jerky, and canned fish like tuna or salmon.

Use protein supplements: Protein supplements like whey protein powder or collagen peptides can also be used to increase protein intake. These can be added to smoothies, shakes, or even coffee to help you meet your daily protein needs.

It is important to note that while protein is important for overall health, too much protein intake can also be harmful to the body. It is recommended to consult with a healthcare professional or registered dietitian to determine the appropriate amount of protein for your individual needs.

CHAPTER SIX

THE ROLE OF VEGETABLES IN THE DIET

Explain the importance of incorporating vegetables into a high-fat, zero-carb, zero-sugar diet for essential nutrients and fiber.

While the high-fat, zero-carb, zero-sugar diet emphasizes consuming high amounts of healthy fats and moderate amounts of protein, it is equally important to incorporate vegetables into the diet to obtain essential nutrients and fiber.

Vegetables are rich in vitamins, minerals, and antioxidants that are necessary for maintaining good health. These nutrients are often lacking in high-fat, low-carb diets that exclude fruits and starchy vegetables. Consuming a variety of vegetables can help prevent nutrient deficiencies and support overall health.

In addition to providing essential nutrients, vegetables are also an excellent source of fiber. Fiber is important for maintaining digestive health, regulating blood sugar levels, and promoting feelings of fullness and satiety. Incorporating non-starchy vegetables, such as leafy greens, broccoli, cauliflower, and peppers, can help individuals following a high-fat, zero-carb, zero-sugar diet obtain the fiber they need.

While the high-fat, zero-carb, zero-sugar diet restricts carbohydrates, it is still important to include non-starchy vegetables in the diet for their essential nutrients and fiber. Vegetables are a great source of vitamins, minerals, and antioxidants that support overall health and well-being. Additionally, fiber from vegetables helps to promote healthy digestion, reduce inflammation, and regulate blood sugar levels.

When choosing vegetables for this diet, it is important to focus on low-carb options such as leafy greens, cruciferous vegetables, and other non-starchy options. Some examples include spinach, kale, broccoli, cauliflower, zucchini, cucumber, and asparagus. These vegetables are also low in calories, making them a great addition to meals and snacks.

To maximize the nutritional value of these vegetables, it is best to prepare them in a way that preserves their nutrients. This can include steaming, sautéing, or roasting them with healthy fats such as olive oil or avocado oil. It is also important to avoid overcooking them, as this can cause a loss of nutrients.

Incorporating vegetables into meals and snacks can be easy and delicious. Adding leafy greens to a smoothie, including roasted vegetables in a salad, or using zucchini noodles as a substitute for traditional pasta are just a few examples. By including a variety of low-carb vegetables in the diet, individuals can reap the benefits of essential nutrients and fiber while maintaining a state of ketosis.

Why Vegetables are Still Important on this Diet

Vegetables are a source of nutrients that cannot be found in other food groups.

Vegetables are a crucial source of nutrients that cannot be found in other food groups. They provide a wide range of essential vitamins, minerals, and fiber that are necessary for optimal health. For example, leafy greens such as kale, spinach, and broccoli are high in vitamin K, which is important for blood clotting and bone health. Carrots, sweet potatoes, and pumpkin are rich in vitamin A, which is necessary for healthy vision, immune function, and skin health. Peppers, tomatoes, and citrus fruits are high in vitamin C, which is important for immune function, collagen production, and wound healing.

Vegetables are also an excellent source of fiber, which plays a crucial role in digestive health and maintaining healthy blood sugar levels. Fiber helps to keep the digestive system functioning properly, promotes feelings of fullness, and can help to lower cholesterol levels. Many low-carb vegetables are high in fiber, including leafy greens, broccoli, cauliflower, Brussels sprouts, and asparagus.

It is important to focus on incorporating a variety of low-carb vegetables into a high-fat, zero-carb, zero-sugar diet to ensure that the body is receiving all the necessary nutrients. Preparing vegetables properly can also maximize their nutritional value. For example, steaming or roasting vegetables can help to retain more nutrients than boiling them. Additionally, pairing vegetables with healthy fats, such as olive oil or avocado, can help the body absorb fat-soluble vitamins found in vegetables.

Vegetables are rich in vitamins A, C, K, and B vitamins, as well as minerals like potassium, magnesium, and calcium.

Vegetables are an excellent source of essential nutrients that are necessary for optimal health. They contain a wide range of vitamins and minerals, including vitamins A, C, K, and B vitamins, as well as minerals like potassium, magnesium, and calcium.

Vitamin A is important for vision, immune function, and skin health, while vitamin C plays a key role in immune function and the growth and repair of tissues. Vitamin K is essential for blood clotting, and the B vitamins help to maintain healthy skin, eyes, and liver function, as well as supporting the nervous system.

Minerals like potassium, magnesium, and calcium are crucial for maintaining strong bones, regulating blood pressure, and supporting muscle and nerve function. These nutrients are essential for overall health and wellbeing and cannot be found in significant amounts in other food groups.

Incorporating a variety of low-carb vegetables into a high-fat, zero-carb, zero-sugar diet is important to ensure that the body is getting a range of essential vitamins and minerals. By doing so, individuals can support optimal health and function at their best.

Vegetable are also an excellent source of fiber, which is essential for gut health and can help regulate blood sugar levels.

Vegetables are an excellent source of dietary fiber, which is a type of carbohydrate that the body cannot digest. Unlike other carbohydrates, fiber passes through the digestive system relatively intact and provides many health benefits.

Fiber plays an important role in maintaining gut health by promoting the growth of healthy gut bacteria and preventing constipation. It can also help regulate blood sugar levels by slowing the absorption of carbohydrates, preventing blood sugar spikes, and promoting insulin sensitivity.

Low-carb vegetables are particularly high in fiber, making them an essential component of a high-fat, zero-carb, zero-sugar diet. Some of the best low-carb vegetables to include are leafy greens, such as spinach, kale, and Swiss chard, as well as cruciferous vegetables like broccoli, cauliflower, and cabbage. These vegetables are also rich in vitamins, minerals, and antioxidants, making them an excellent source of essential nutrients that cannot be found in other food groups.

To maximize the nutritional value of vegetables, it's important to prepare them in a way that preserves their nutrients. Steaming, roasting, or sautéing vegetables lightly can help preserve their vitamin and mineral content. Additionally, adding healthy fats like olive oil, avocado, or nuts to vegetables can help the body absorb fat-soluble vitamins like vitamin A, D, E, and K.

Vegetables contain phytochemicals, which have anti-inflammatory and antioxidant effects, and can reduce the risk of chronic diseases.

Certain vegetables contain phytochemicals, which are natural compounds that give plants their color, flavor, and smell. These compounds have been found to have a range of health benefits, including anti-inflammatory and antioxidant effects. For example, cruciferous vegetables like broccoli and kale contain sulforaphane, which has been shown to reduce inflammation and may even have anti-cancer properties. Similarly, tomatoes contain lycopene, which has been linked to a reduced risk of heart disease and certain types of cancer.

Eating a variety of vegetables can ensure that the body is getting a range of phytochemicals, which can help reduce the risk of chronic diseases. In addition to their phytochemical content, vegetables are also rich in essential vitamins, minerals, and fiber, making them an important part of any healthy diet, including a high-fat, zero-carb, zero-sugar diet.

Best Low-Carb Vegetables to Include in Meals

There are many low-carb vegetables that can be included in meals on this diet.

When following a high-fat, zero-carb, zero-sugar diet, it is still possible to include a variety of low-carb vegetables in meals. In fact, incorporating low-carb vegetables into the diet can provide a range of essential nutrients and fiber that may not be obtained from other food groups.

Some examples of low-carb vegetables include leafy greens such as spinach, kale, and lettuce, cruciferous vegetables such as broccoli, cauliflower, and cabbage, and other vegetables such as zucchini, bell peppers, and asparagus. These vegetables are also rich in vitamins and minerals, such as vitamin C, vitamin K, potassium, and magnesium.

To maximize the nutritional value of vegetables, it is important to prepare them in a way that retains their nutrients. Cooking methods like boiling and frying can cause vegetables to lose some of their nutrient content, while steaming and sautéing can help to preserve their nutrients. It is also important to avoid adding high-carb ingredients like sauces or bread crumbs to vegetable dishes.

By incorporating a variety of low-carb vegetables into meals, individuals on this diet can still obtain the essential nutrients and fiber needed for optimal health.

Low-carb vegetables, including leafy greens, cruciferous vegetables, cucumbers, bell peppers, mushrooms, zucchini, summer squashes, and asparagus.

Here is a list of some of the best low-carb vegetables that can be incorporated into a high-fat, zero-carb, zero-sugar diet:

- **Leafy greens:** spinach, kale, collard greens, Swiss chard, arugula, and lettuce.
- **Cruciferous vegetables:** broccoli, cauliflower, Brussels sprouts, and cabbage.
- **Cucumbers:** both regular and English cucumbers are low in carbs and high in water content.

- ➢ **Bell peppers:** red, green, and yellow bell peppers are low in carbs and high in vitamin C.
- ➢ **Mushrooms:** low in carbs and high in antioxidants and minerals like potassium.
- ➢ **Zucchini:** a versatile vegetable that can be used in a variety of dishes, low in carbs and high in fiber.
- ➢ **Summer squashes:** yellow squash, pattypan squash, and zucchini are all low in carbs and high in vitamins and minerals.
- ➢ **Asparagus:** a low-carb vegetable that is high in fiber, vitamins A, C, E, and K, as well as folate.

These vegetables can be prepared in various ways, such as roasted, sautéed, grilled, or eaten raw in salads. By incorporating these low-carb vegetables into meals, one can ensure that they are getting a variety of essential nutrients and fiber that are important for overall health.

Starchy vegetables should be avoided.

Starchy vegetables such as potatoes, sweet potatoes, yams, and corn are high in carbohydrates and can significantly impact blood sugar levels. These vegetables contain high amounts of starch, which is a type of carbohydrate that breaks down quickly into glucose, leading to spikes in blood sugar levels. Additionally, starchy vegetables are often high in calories, which can make it more difficult to achieve weight loss goals on a high-fat, zero-carb, zero-sugar diet. Therefore, it is generally recommended to avoid starchy vegetables on this type of diet to ensure the body stays in a state of ketosis and to maintain stable blood sugar levels.

How to Prepare Vegetables to Maximize Their Nutritional Value

The importance of preparing vegetables in a way that preserves their nutrients.

The way that vegetables are prepared can have a significant impact on their nutrient content. Overcooking or boiling vegetables for extended periods can lead to nutrient loss, particularly water-soluble vitamins like vitamin C and B vitamins. It is therefore important to use methods of cooking that preserve as many of the nutrients as possible.

One effective way to preserve nutrients in vegetables is to steam them. Steaming helps to retain the water-soluble vitamins and minerals that would otherwise be lost during boiling. Roasting or grilling vegetables can also be a good option, as this can help to caramelize the natural sugars in the vegetables and give them a delicious flavor without the need for added fats or sugars.

It's also essential to avoid overcooking vegetables, as this can lead to the breakdown of the cell walls, making them mushy and devoid of nutrients. Vegetables should be cooked until they are just tender but still have some crunch.

In addition to cooking methods, it's also important to store vegetables correctly to ensure that they retain their nutrients. Storing vegetables in a cool, dry place or in the refrigerator can help to slow down the breakdown of nutrients and preserve their freshness. Overall, the preparation and storage of vegetables play a vital role in maximizing their nutritional value and ensuring that they provide the body with the essential nutrients it needs.

When preparing vegetables on a high-fat, zero-carb, zero-sugar diet, it's important to keep in mind that certain cooking methods can lead to nutrient loss. Overcooking or boiling vegetables for extended periods can result in the loss of essential nutrients such as vitamins and minerals.

To maximize the nutritional value of vegetables, it's best to lightly steam or sauté them in healthy fats such as olive oil or coconut oil. Pairing vegetables with healthy fats not only enhances their flavor but also helps to increase the absorption of fat-soluble vitamins such as vitamins A, D, E, and K.

Incorporating herbs and spices can also add flavor and nutrients to vegetables without adding extra calories or carbs. Some examples of nutrient-rich herbs and spices include basil, parsley, cilantro, garlic, ginger, and turmeric.

Fermented vegetables such as sauerkraut, kimchi, and pickles are also a great addition to a high-fat, zero-carb, zero-sugar diet. Fermented vegetables are rich in probiotics, which can help to support gut health and boost the immune system.

Overall, the key to preparing vegetables on this diet is to keep it simple, experiment with different cooking methods and flavorings, and choose nutrient-dense vegetables that are low in carbs.

Steaming, roasting, and sautéing are good cooking methods to preserve the nutrient content of vegetables.

Steaming is a gentle cooking method that helps to preserve the color, texture, and flavor of vegetables. To steam vegetables, place them in a steamer basket or colander over a pot of boiling water and cover with a lid. Cook until tender but still slightly firm.

Roasting is a great way to bring out the natural sweetness and flavor of vegetables. To roast vegetables, toss them with a little oil and seasonings and spread them out in a single layer on a baking sheet. Roast in a preheated oven until tender and lightly browned.

Sautéing is a quick and easy way to cook vegetables while retaining their nutrients and flavor. To sauté vegetables, heat a little oil in a pan over medium-high heat, add the vegetables, and cook until tender and lightly browned, stirring occasionally.

It's important to avoid overcooking vegetables, as this can lead to a loss of nutrients. Pairing vegetables with healthy fats, such as olive oil or avocado, can also help to increase the absorption of fat-soluble vitamins. Experimenting with herbs and spices can add flavor without adding extra calories or salt. Lastly, incorporating fermented vegetables, such as sauerkraut or kimchi, can provide additional health benefits by promoting gut health.

Incorporating low-carb vegetables into a high-fat, zero-carb, zero-sugar diet is crucial for obtaining essential nutrients and fiber that cannot be found in other food groups. Vegetables are rich in vitamins A, C, K, and B vitamins, as well as minerals like potassium, magnesium, and calcium. They are also an excellent source of fiber, which is essential for gut health and can help regulate blood sugar levels. Certain vegetables contain phytochemicals that have anti-inflammatory and antioxidant effects, reducing the risk of chronic diseases. The best low-carb vegetables to include in meals include leafy greens, cruciferous vegetables, cucumbers, bell peppers, mushrooms, zucchini, summer squ

CHAPTER SEVEN

MEAL PLANNING AND RECIPES

Importance of meal planning and recipes in a high-fat, zero-carb, zero-sugar diet

Meal planning and recipes play a crucial role in a high-fat, zero-carb, zero-sugar diet. This is because the diet requires careful planning to ensure that meals are nutritionally balanced and satisfying, while also adhering to the principles of the diet.

One of the most important aspects of meal planning is ensuring that meals contain enough healthy fats and protein while keeping carbohydrates to a minimum. This requires careful selection of foods and ingredients, as well as portion control.

Recipes designed specifically for this diet can be helpful in providing guidance and inspiration for meal planning. They can also help to ensure that meals are tasty and varied, which is important for long-term adherence to the diet.

When planning meals and selecting recipes, it's important to prioritize whole, unprocessed foods and avoid highly processed, low-nutrient options. This ensures that meals are nutrient-dense and provide the body with the essential vitamins, minerals, and other nutrients it needs to function properly.

It's also important to plan for snacks and on-the-go meals, as these can be challenging on a high-fat, zero-carb, zero-sugar diet. Portable, low-carb snacks such as nuts, seeds, and hard-boiled eggs can be a good option.

Overall, meal planning and recipes are essential components of a successful high-fat, zero-carb, zero-sugar diet. With careful planning and attention to nutrition, this diet can provide a wide range of health benefits and promote long-term health and wellness.

Here are some tips to make meal planning and preparation second nature in a high-fat, zero-carb, zero-sugar diet:

- **Set a regular schedule**: Set aside time each week to plan out your meals and grocery list. Consistency is key in making meal planning and preparation a habit.

- **Plan for leftovers:** Plan meals that will produce leftovers that can be easily reheated for a quick and easy meal the next day.

- **Keep it simple:** Focus on meals that are easy to prepare and require minimal ingredients. Simple meals can still be flavorful and nutritious.

- **Batch cook:** Prepare large batches of food, such as roasted vegetables or grilled chicken, to use throughout the week in different meals.

- **Use recipes:** Look for recipes that fit your dietary restrictions and use them as a guide for meal planning and preparation. This can help take the guesswork out of meal planning and ensure a variety of flavors and nutrients.

- **Stock up on staples:** Keep your pantry and fridge stocked with staples like low-carb vegetables, healthy fats, and protein sources, so you always have the building blocks for a meal on hand.

➢ **Prep ahead:** Prepping ingredients ahead of time, like chopping vegetables or marinating meat, can save time during meal preparation.

By incorporating these tips into your routine, meal planning and preparation can become second nature and make following a high-fat, zero-carb, zero-sugar diet much easier.

Sample meal plans for different calorie levels
Here are sample meal plans for a high-fat, zero-carb, zero-sugar diet for different calorie levels:

1200 Calorie Meal Plan:
Here's a sample 1200 calorie meal plan for a high-fat, zero-carb, zero-sugar diet:

Breakfast:

Scrambled eggs with spinach and mushrooms cooked in coconut oil
1 small avocado
Snack:

1 ounce of almonds
Lunch:

Grilled chicken breast on a bed of mixed greens with olive oil and vinegar dressing
Roasted asparagus spears
Snack:

1 ounce of cheddar cheese
Dinner:

Baked salmon with a side of steamed broccoli and cauliflower, topped with butter and garlic

Note: This meal plan is for illustrative purposes only and should not be followed without consulting a healthcare professional. The number of calories required per day varies depending on factors such as age, gender, height, weight, and activity level.

1500 Calorie Meal Plan:
Here is a sample 1500 calorie meal plan for a high-fat, zero-carb, zero-sugar diet:

Breakfast:

Two eggs cooked in coconut oil
1/2 avocado
1/4 cup cherry tomatoes
Black coffee or tea with unsweetened almond milk
Snack:

Celery sticks with almond butter
Lunch:

Grilled chicken breast
1 cup of mixed leafy greens
1/4 cup of sliced cucumbers
1/4 cup of sliced bell peppers
Olive oil and apple cider vinegar dressing
Snack:

A handful of macadamia nuts
Dinner:

Grilled salmon fillet

1 cup of roasted asparagus
1/4 cup of roasted mushrooms
1/2 cup of cauliflower rice cooked in coconut oil

1800 Calorie Meal Plan:
Here's a sample 1800 calorie meal plan for a high-fat, zero-carb, zero-sugar diet:

Breakfast:

2 scrambled eggs cooked in butter or coconut oil
2 strips of bacon
1 cup of spinach sautéed in olive oil
Snack:

1 oz of almonds
1 hard-boiled egg
Lunch:

4 oz of grilled chicken breast
1/2 avocado
1 cup of mixed greens topped with olive oil and balsamic vinegar dressing
Snack:

2 celery stalks with 2 tablespoons of almond butter
Dinner:

6 oz of salmon cooked in butter or coconut oil
1 cup of roasted broccoli and cauliflower
1/2 cup of sautéed mushrooms in olive oil

Remember to adjust portion sizes according to individual needs and to consult with a healthcare professional before making any major changes to your diet.

Recipes for breakfast, lunch, dinner, and snacks for the high-fat, zero-carb, zero-sugar diet

Sure, here are some recipe ideas for each meal and snacks:

Breakfast:
- Keto pancakes made with almond flour, eggs, and cream cheese
- Scrambled eggs with avocado and bacon
- Keto smoothie bowl made with coconut milk, spinach, avocado, and almond butter
- Chia seed pudding made with coconut milk and topped with berries and nuts

Snacks:
- **Celery sticks with almond butter**
- **Hard-boiled eggs**
- **Beef jerky**
- **Cheese cubes with olives**

Lunch:

- Greek salad with mixed greens, cucumber, cherry tomatoes, feta cheese, and olives with olive oil and lemon dressing
- Grilled chicken breast with roasted Brussels sprouts and cauliflower rice
- Tuna salad made with avocado, mayo, celery, and dill, served with lettuce cups
- Zucchini noodles with pesto sauce and grilled shrimp

Snacks:
- Keto fat bombs made with coconut oil, cocoa powder, and nuts

> Sliced cucumber with hummus
> Pork rinds
> Sugar-free jello

Dinner:
> Grilled salmon with asparagus and cauliflower mash
> Beef stir-fry with broccoli, bell peppers, and mushrooms
> Keto pizza made with cauliflower crust, tomato sauce, cheese, and toppings of choice
> Stuffed bell peppers with ground beef, cauliflower rice, and tomato sauce

Snacks:
> Roasted almonds with sea salt
> Keto protein shake made with almond milk, protein powder, and coconut oil
> Cheese crisps made with shredded cheese baked in the oven
> Smoked salmon with cream cheese on cucumber slices

Note: The serving sizes and proportions of macronutrients may vary based on individual dietary needs and goals. It's important to consult with a healthcare professional or registered dietitian before making significant changes to your diet.

Breakfast recipes:
> Bacon and Eggs
> Keto Pancakes
> Greek Yogurt and Berries

Here are three recipes for breakfast on the high-fat, zero-carb, zero-sugar diet:

Bacon and Eggs

Ingredients:

- 2-3 strips of bacon
- 2 large eggs
- Salt and pepper to taste

Instructions:

- In a frying pan, cook the bacon until crispy. Remove from the pan and set aside.
- Crack the eggs into the pan with the bacon fat and cook to your desired doneness. Season with salt and pepper.
- Serve the eggs with the bacon on the side.

Keto Pancakes

Ingredients:

- 2 eggs
- 1/4 cup almond flour
- 1/4 cup cream cheese, softened
- 1/4 tsp baking powder
- 1/4 tsp vanilla extract
- Butter or coconut oil for frying

Instructions:

- In a mixing bowl, whisk together the eggs, almond flour, cream cheese, baking powder, and vanilla extract until smooth.
- Heat a frying pan over medium heat and add butter or coconut oil to the pan.
- Spoon the pancake batter into the pan and cook for 2-3 minutes on each side or until golden brown.
- Serve with butter and sugar-free syrup if desired.

Greek Yogurt and Berries

Ingredients:

- 1/2 cup plain Greek yogurt

> 1/4 cup mixed berries (strawberries, raspberries, blueberries)

Instructions:
> Spoon the Greek yogurt into a bowl.
> Top with mixed berries and enjoy!

Note: Make sure to check the label of the Greek yogurt to ensure it is low in carbs and free of added sugars.

Lunch recipes:
> Chicken Caesar Salad
> Tuna Salad
> Cauliflower Fried Rice

Here are the recipes for the mentioned lunch options:

Chicken Caesar Salad:
> 4 oz. grilled chicken breast
> 2 cups chopped romaine lettuce
> 2 tbsp Caesar dressing (made with healthy fats like olive oil or avocado oil)
> 2 tbsp grated parmesan cheese
> Salt and pepper to taste

Instructions:
> Season the chicken breast with salt and pepper and grill until cooked through.
> Chop the romaine lettuce and place in a bowl.
> Add the cooked chicken to the bowl and toss with Caesar dressing.
> Top with grated parmesan cheese.

Tuna Salad:
> 5 oz. can of tuna in water, drained
> 2 tbsp mayonnaise (made with healthy oils like avocado or olive oil)

- ➢ 1 tbsp Dijon mustard
- ➢ 1 celery stalk, diced
- ➢ 1 small dill pickle, diced
- ➢ Salt and pepper to taste

Instructions:
- ➢ In a small bowl, combine the drained tuna, mayonnaise, Dijon mustard, celery, and pickle.
- ➢ Mix well and season with salt and pepper to taste.
- ➢ Serve on a bed of lettuce or wrapped in lettuce leaves.

Cauliflower Fried Rice:
- ➢ 1 head of cauliflower, riced
- ➢ 2 tbsp coconut oil
- ➢ 1 onion, diced
- ➢ 2 garlic cloves, minced
- ➢ 1 cup chopped mixed vegetables (carrots, peas, and bell peppers work well)
- ➢ 2 eggs, beaten
- ➢ 2 tbsp soy sauce or coconut aminos
- ➢ Salt and pepper to taste

Instructions:
- ➢ Heat the coconut oil in a large skillet over medium heat.
- ➢ Add the onion and garlic and sauté until softened.
- ➢ Add the mixed vegetables and continue to sauté until tender.
- ➢ Push the vegetables to one side of the pan and add the beaten eggs to the other side.
- ➢ Scramble the eggs until cooked through and then mix with the vegetables.
- ➢ Add the riced cauliflower to the skillet and stir to combine.
- ➢ Drizzle with soy sauce or coconut aminos and season with salt and pepper to taste. Cook for an additional 5-10 minutes until the cauliflower is tender.

Dinner recipes:

> ➢ Grilled Steak and Asparagus
> ➢ Zucchini Noodle Lasagna
> ➢ Salmon with Roasted Vegetables

Grilled Steak and Asparagus Recipe:

Ingredients:
> ➢ 1 lb flank steak
> ➢ 1 lb asparagus
> ➢ 1 tbsp olive oil
> ➢ 1 tsp garlic powder
> ➢ 1 tsp dried rosemary
> ➢ Salt and pepper to taste

Instructions:
> ➢ Preheat grill to medium-high heat.
> ➢ Season the steak with garlic powder, dried rosemary, salt, and pepper.
> ➢ Brush the asparagus with olive oil and season with salt and pepper.
> ➢ Place the steak on the grill and cook for 4-5 minutes on each side, or until desired doneness is reached.
> ➢ Remove the steak from the grill and let it rest for 5-10 minutes.
> ➢ Place the asparagus on the grill and cook for 3-4 minutes, or until slightly charred and tender.
> ➢ Slice the steak against the grain and serve with the grilled asparagus.

Zucchini Noodle Lasagna Recipe:

Ingredients:
> ➢ 4 medium zucchinis, sliced lengthwise into thin noodles
> ➢ 1 lb ground beef
> ➢ 1 jar low-sugar marinara sauce
> ➢ 2 cups ricotta cheese
> ➢ 1 egg

- ➢ 1 tsp dried basil
- ➢ 1 tsp dried oregano
- ➢ Salt and pepper to taste
- ➢ 1 cup shredded mozzarella cheese

Instructions:

- ➢ Preheat oven to 375°F.
- ➢ In a large skillet, cook the ground beef over medium heat until browned.
- ➢ Add the marinara sauce to the skillet and stir to combine.
- ➢ In a separate bowl, mix together the ricotta cheese, egg, basil, oregano, salt, and pepper.
- ➢ Layer the zucchini noodles, meat sauce, and ricotta mixture in a 9x13 inch baking dish.
- ➢ Repeat the layering process until all ingredients are used, ending with a layer of meat sauce.
- ➢ Top with shredded mozzarella cheese.
- ➢ Bake for 35-40 minutes, or until the cheese is melted and bubbly.

Salmon with Roasted Vegetables Recipe:

Ingredients:

- ➢ 4 salmon fillets
- ➢ 1 lb brussels sprouts, trimmed and halved
- ➢ 1 lb carrots, peeled and cut into 1-inch pieces
- ➢ 1 red onion, cut into wedges
- ➢ 3 tbsp olive oil
- ➢ 1 tsp garlic powder
- ➢ 1 tsp dried thyme
- ➢ Salt and pepper to taste

Instructions:

- ➢ Preheat oven to 400°F.
- ➢ In a large bowl, toss the brussels sprouts, carrots, and red onion with olive oil, garlic powder, thyme, salt, and pepper.

- ➤ Spread the vegetables out on a large baking sheet and roast for 20-25 minutes, or until tender and slightly charred.
- ➤ Season the salmon fillets with salt and pepper.
- ➤ Place the salmon on the baking sheet with the vegetables.
- ➤ Return the baking sheet to the oven and roast for an additional 10-12 minutes, or until the salmon is cooked through and flaky.

Snack recipes:
- ➤ Cheese and Nuts
- ➤ Guacamole with Veggies
- ➤ Chocolate Fat Bombs

Here are some recipes for high-fat, zero-carb, zero-sugar snacks:

- ➤ **Cheese and Nuts:** This simple snack is perfect for when you're on the go or just need something quick and easy. Simply grab a serving of your favorite cheese, such as cheddar or brie, and pair it with a handful of almonds, macadamia nuts, or walnuts.

- ➤ **Guacamole with Veggies:** Guacamole is a delicious and healthy snack that's high in healthy fats. To make it, mash together 1 ripe avocado with 1 tablespoon of lime juice and a pinch of salt. Serve with sliced vegetables like bell peppers, cucumbers, and carrots for dipping.

- ➤ **Chocolate Fat Bombs:** These decadent treats are perfect for satisfying a sweet tooth while sticking to a high-fat, low-carb diet. To make them, combine 1/2 cup coconut oil, 1/2 cup almond butter, 1/4 cup unsweetened cocoa powder, and a pinch of salt. Spoon the mixture into a silicone mold and freeze until solid. Store in the freezer for a quick and easy snack.

Remember, it's important to choose snacks that are high in healthy fats and low in carbs and sugar to stay on track with your high-fat, zero-carb, zero-sugar diet.

Modifying favorite recipes to fit the high-fat, zero-carb, zero-sugar diet.

Importance of modifying recipes to fit dietary needs.

Modifying recipes to fit dietary needs is essential for individuals who are following a high-fat, zero-carb, zero-sugar diet, or any other dietary restrictions. It is important to adjust the ingredients used in a recipe to ensure that the dish is compliant with the dietary guidelines.

By modifying recipes, individuals can ensure that they are consuming the necessary macronutrients and micronutrients without compromising taste and flavor. For example, traditional recipes that use wheat flour for baking can be modified to use almond flour or coconut flour, which are low-carb and high-fat alternatives.

Additionally, individuals can modify the amount of sugar used in a recipe or use sugar substitutes like stevia or erythritol, which do not affect blood sugar levels. This allows individuals to still enjoy sweet treats without consuming excess carbs or sugar.

Modifying recipes to fit dietary needs also allows for more variety in meal options and can prevent boredom with the same foods. It also provides individuals with the opportunity to be creative in the kitchen and experiment with new ingredients and flavors.

Overall, modifying recipes is a crucial aspect of following a high-fat, zero-carb, zero-sugar diet or any other dietary restriction, as it allows individuals to tailor their meals to meet their specific nutritional needs while still enjoying tasty and satisfying food.

Tips on modifying recipes.

Modifying recipes to fit dietary needs can be challenging, but with some simple tips, it can be done successfully. **Here are some tips for modifying recipes:**

> **Understand the basics of the diet:** Before modifying a recipe, it is essential to understand the basics of the high-fat, zero-carb, zero-sugar diet. This will help in making the right substitutions and modifications.

> **Substitute high-carb ingredients**: Identify the high-carb ingredients in the recipe and substitute them with low-carb alternatives. For example, instead of using regular flour, use almond flour or coconut flour.

> **Use healthy fats:** Incorporate healthy fats into the recipe to increase the fat content. Use olive oil, coconut oil, butter, or ghee instead of vegetable oils.

> **Adjust seasoning and spices:** Adjust the seasoning and spices to suit your taste buds. Experiment with different herbs and spices to add flavor without adding carbs.

> **Check nutrition information:** Use a nutrition calculator to check the nutritional information of the recipe after making modifications. This will help in ensuring that the recipe is still in line with the dietary needs.

- **Keep it simple:** Keep the recipe simple and avoid using too many ingredients. This will make it easier to modify the recipe and ensure that it still tastes delicious.

- **Be creative:** Be creative with substitutions and modifications. Experiment with different ingredients and find what works best for you.

Overall, modifying recipes can be a fun and creative process that can help you enjoy your favorite foods while still following your dietary needs.

Examples of recipe modifications

Sure, here are a few examples of recipe modifications:

- **Substitute high-carb ingredients:** You can substitute high-carb ingredients with low-carb alternatives. For example, if a recipe calls for flour, you can use almond flour or coconut flour instead.

- **Replace sugar with a sugar substitute:** Sugar is not allowed in a zero-sugar diet, but you can use sugar substitutes like stevia or erythritol.

- **Use healthy fats:** Replace unhealthy fats like vegetable oils with healthy fats like coconut oil, olive oil, or avocado oil.

- **Increase protein content**: If you need more protein in your diet, you can add extra protein to a recipe by using protein powder or adding extra meat or tofu.

- **Adjust portion sizes:** If a recipe has too many carbs or calories for your needs, you can adjust the portion sizes or make fewer servings.

> **Experiment with herbs and spices**: You can use herbs and spices to add flavor to a recipe without adding extra carbs or calories. Try using fresh herbs like basil, rosemary, or thyme, or spices like cumin, chili powder, or paprika.

> **Add vegetables:** Adding vegetables to a recipe is an easy way to increase the nutrient content and add fiber without adding extra carbs. Try adding leafy greens, broccoli, or cauliflower to soups, stews, or casseroles.

CHAPTER EIGHT

MAINTAINING THE DIET LONG-TERM

The high-fat, zero-carb, zero-sugar diet can be challenging to maintain long-term.

The high-fat, zero-carb, zero-sugar diet can be challenging to maintain long-term due to its strict dietary restrictions and potential for nutrient deficiencies. While the diet may be effective for weight loss and managing certain health conditions, it is important to consider the potential drawbacks and long-term sustainability.

One challenge of the high-fat, zero-carb, zero-sugar diet is the limited food options, which can make it difficult to adhere to the diet long-term. Additionally, the high-fat nature of the diet may be difficult for some people to tolerate, leading to gastrointestinal discomfort.

Another potential issue is nutrient deficiencies, particularly in vitamins and minerals commonly found in fruits, whole grains, and legumes. It is important to ensure adequate intake of essential nutrients through careful meal planning and, if necessary, supplementation.

Finally, social situations can also be challenging on this diet, as it may be difficult to find suitable options when dining out or attending events.

To maintain the high-fat, zero-carb, zero-sugar diet long-term, it is important to have a solid understanding of the dietary restrictions and to plan meals carefully to ensure adequate nutrient intake. It may also be helpful to seek support from a healthcare provider or registered dietitian to address any potential nutrient deficiencies and to develop a sustainable eating plan.

The high-fat, zero-carb, zero-sugar diet can be challenging to maintain long-term, as it requires a significant shift in dietary habits and a commitment to avoiding certain foods. However, with proper planning and dedication, it is possible to stick to this diet and reap its benefits.

One key to long-term success on this diet is meal planning. By planning out meals and snacks ahead of time, it becomes easier to stick to the diet and avoid temptations to eat non-compliant foods. It is also important to have a variety of meal options to avoid getting bored with the diet.

Another strategy for long-term success is to find support from others who are also following this diet. This could include joining a support group or finding an accountability partner who can offer encouragement and help keep you on track.

It is also important to remember that while this diet can be effective for weight loss and improving overall health, it may not be suitable for everyone. It is important to consult with a healthcare professional before starting any new diet, especially if you have pre-existing health conditions.

In summary, the high-fat, zero-carb, zero-sugar diet can be challenging to maintain long-term, but with proper planning, dedication, and support, it is possible to stick to this diet and reap its benefits. As with any diet, it is important to consult with a healthcare professional before starting and to listen to your body's needs.

Strategies for Maintaining the High-Fat, Zero-Carb, Zero-Sugar Diet

Plan Ahead

Planning is one of the most important aspects of maintaining a high-fat, zero-carb, zero-sugar diet. Without proper planning, it can be challenging to stick to the diet and find suitable options when hunger strikes.

One of the best ways to plan is to create a meal plan for the week or month. This meal plan should include all meals and snacks and consider the individual's calorie and nutrient needs. It's essential to incorporate a variety of low-carb vegetables, healthy fats, and protein sources.

When creating a meal plan, it's also crucial to consider potential obstacles that could derail the diet. For example, if the individual has a busy week ahead, it may be necessary to prep meals and snacks in advance or plan for quick and easy options.

Another way to plan is to create a grocery list before going to the store. This list should include all the ingredients needed for the planned meals and snacks, as well as any staples that may be needed for cooking and meal prep.

Planning can also help avoid temptation when dining out or attending social events. By researching menus and planning, it's possible to find suitable options that fit within the diet's guidelines.

Overall, planning is crucial for maintaining a high-fat, zero-carb, zero-sugar diet long-term. It helps ensure that the individual stays on track and always has suitable options available.

Find Support

Finding support is an essential part of sticking to the high-fat, zero-carb, zero-sugar diet. It can be challenging to make dietary changes on your own, so seeking support from others who are also following this diet can be helpful. **Here are some ways to find support:**

> ➤ **Join a support group:** There are many online communities and forums dedicated to the high-fat, zero-carb, zero-sugar diet. Joining a support group can provide you with a sense of community and accountability, as well as a place to ask questions and share experiences.

> ➤ **Find a buddy:** Having a friend or family member who is also following the same diet can be beneficial. You can share recipes, meal plans, and motivation to help each other stay on track.

> ➤ **Work with a dietitian:** A registered dietitian who is knowledgeable about the high-fat, zero-carb, zero-sugar diet can provide you with personalized guidance and support. They can help you create meal plans, navigate food choices, and address any concerns or challenges you may encounter.

> ➤ **Seek professional counseling**: Making dietary changes can be challenging, and it can be helpful to talk to a mental health professional if you are struggling. They can provide you with support and strategies for managing any emotional or psychological barriers to sticking to the diet.

By finding support, you can increase your chances of sticking to the high-fat, zero-carb, zero-sugar diet long-term and achieving your health goals.

When following a high-fat, zero-carb, zero-sugar diet, it's important to focus on whole, nutrient-dense foods. These are foods that provide a high level of nutrients per calorie and are minimally processed. **Some examples of nutrient-dense foods that can be incorporated into this diet include:**

- ➢ **Low-carb vegetables:** As mentioned earlier, vegetables are an important source of fiber, vitamins, and minerals, and many are low in carbohydrates. Focus on leafy greens, cruciferous vegetables, cucumbers, bell peppers, mushrooms, zucchini, summer squashes, and asparagus.

- ➢ **Healthy fats:** This diet is high in fat, but it's important to choose healthy sources of fat. Some examples include avocado, olive oil, coconut oil, nuts, seeds, and fatty fish.

- ➢ **Protein sources:** Choose high-quality sources of protein, such as grass-fed beef, wild-caught fish, free-range poultry, and eggs.

- ➢ **Berries:** While most fruits are high in carbohydrates, berries are a good low-carb option that are also high in antioxidants and fiber.

- ➢ **Fermented foods:** These foods, such as sauerkraut and kimchi, are a good source of probiotics, which can help promote a healthy gut microbiome.

- ➢ **Herbs and spices:** Using herbs and spices in cooking can add flavor and nutrition to meals.

By focusing on whole, nutrient-dense foods, this diet can provide a wide range of nutrients while still being low in carbohydrates and sugar.

Address Social Situations

Addressing social situations can be one of the biggest challenges when following a high-fat, zero-carb, zero-sugar diet. **Here are some tips to help navigate social situations:**

> **Plan ahead:** If you know you will be attending an event or gathering where food will be served, plan ahead. Consider bringing your own dish that fits within your dietary needs, or reach out to the host ahead of time to inquire about the menu and see if there are any modifications that can be made.

> **Be confident in your choices:** When eating out or at a social gathering, be confident in your dietary choices and communicate them clearly to those around you. You can also provide education and information about the benefits of the diet if others are curious or questioning your choices.

> **Focus on socializing:** Remember that social gatherings are not just about the food, but also about spending time with friends and loved ones. Focus on enjoying the company and conversation, rather than solely on the food.

> **Look for healthy options:** When eating out or attending events, look for healthy options that fit within your dietary needs. This may require some creativity or modifications, but many restaurants and caterers are willing to accommodate dietary restrictions.

> **Don't be too hard on yourself**: It's important to remember that following a high-fat, zero-carb, zero-sugar diet can be challenging, and there may be times when it's not possible to stick to your dietary plan. Don't be too hard on yourself and remember that one slip-up does not have to derail your progress. Just get back on track

as soon as possible and continue moving forward with your dietary goals.

Incorporate Occasional Treats

While the high-fat, zero-carb, zero-sugar diet emphasizes whole, nutrient-dense foods, occasional treats can be included in moderation. It is important to choose treats that are low in carbs and sugar, but still satisfy cravings. **Some examples of occasional treats on this diet include:**

> **Dark chocolate:** Choose chocolate that is at least 70% cocoa and low in added sugar.

> **Berries:** Berries are relatively low in carbs and sugar and can be enjoyed as a sweet snack.

> **Nut butter:** Choose natural nut butter that is low in added sugar and can be spread on low-carb crackers or celery.

> **Cheese:** Cheese is a good source of protein and fat and can be a satisfying snack or addition to a meal.

It is important to remember that treats should be enjoyed in moderation and not used as a regular part of the diet. Planning and finding healthy alternatives to high-carb, high-sugar treats can help to stay on track with the diet while still satisfying cravings.

CONCLUSION

In conclusion, the H0 diet can be a beneficial way of eating for some people, but it requires careful planning and dedication to maintain long-term. Incorporating low-carb vegetables, healthy fats, and nutrient-dense foods is essential for meeting daily nutritional needs and avoiding potential deficiencies. Meal planning and preparation can make following this diet easier, and recipe modifications can help accommodate individual dietary needs and preferences. Finding support and addressing social situations can also be helpful in sticking to this diet. Remember, it's essential to listen to your body and adjust as necessary to ensure a healthy and sustainable way of eating.